# Morning Yoga Stretches

*How to Unlock the Full Power of The Best Morning Stretches to Command Your Days and Transform Your Life*

*Morning Yoga Stretches*

# Introduction

*Do you struggle to get through your morning routine without feeling grumpy? Perhaps you have to jumpstart your mind with that cup of coffee, but that is starting to make you caffeine-dependent, which you feel is not healthy for you.*

*Or do you normally feel less energized and rested in the mornings and are now looking for a way to kickstart your day feeling both physically and mentally healthy?*

Well, if that is you, you are not alone.

According to statistics[1] by the New York Post published in May 2020, more than 60% of US citizens cannot say they had enough rest or energy by the time they wake up, which leads to lower motivation, focus, and poor decision-making throughout the day.

But that does not have to be your story every day because I have good news for you! You can rejuvenate your mind and

---

[1] https://nypost.com/2020/05/27/more-than-60-percent-of-americans-rarely-feel-rested-and-energized-in-the-morning/

body as well as get ready for tasks by engaging in some revitalizing yoga stretches

But, even with the assurance that yoga stretches are great, you may still be wondering:

- *Are yoga stretches enough to me you going?*
- *What other benefits of doing yoga can I enjoy?*
- *Are there any side effects of doing yoga?*
- *Can I perform yoga stretches from anywhere?*

And much more.

If you have these and other similar questions, this Morning Yoga Stretches Guide will answer any questions regarding yoga stretches and enlighten you on how to perform them. More specifically, this book will cover subjects like:

- *What yoga is*
- *The origin of yoga*
- *Health benefits of yoga*
- *Tips to get you started on yoga poses*
- *Yoga stretches for different body parts*

*Morning Yoga Stretches*

And much more!

So, if you have ever wondered what this age-old practice can do for your well-being, this is just the book for you!

Shall we begin?


PS: I'd like your feedback. If you are happy with this book, please leave a review on Amazon.

Please leave a review for this book on Amazon by visiting the page below:

https://amzn.to/2VMR5qr

# Table of Content

**Introduction** _____ 2

**Chapter 1: Understanding Yoga and Its Benefits** _____ 11

What Is Yoga? _____ 11

The Origin Of Yoga and Its Evolution _____ 11

What Are The Health Benefits Of Yoga? _____ 12

Can You Do Yoga From Home? _____ 19

**Chapter 2: Breathing and Letting Go During Yoga Stretches** _____ 21

Yoga Breathing Patterns _____ 21

How to Breathe During Yoga _____ 23

How To Let Go _____ 25

**Chapter 3: Tips To Get You Started With Your Morning Yoga Routine** _____ 29

**Chapter 3: Basic Yoga Warm-Up Stretches 36**

Warm-up 1: Child's Pose _____ 36

Warm-up 2: Hero pose _____ 38

Warm-up 3: Wide-leg Stretch _____ 40

Warm-up 4: Cat and Cow _____ 42

Warm-up 5: Up and Down Hands Motion ____ 43

Warm-up 6: Neck Rotations _____ 44

Warm-up 7: Fish Pose _____ 45

Warm-up 8: Tree Pose _____ 47

Warm-up 9: Easy Pose _____ 49

Warm-up 10: Staff Pose _____ 50

## Chapter 4: Morning Yoga Stretches For The Back _____ 51

Bridge Bends _____ 51

Seated Forward Yoga Bend _____ 53

Head-to-Knee Forward Bend _____ 55

Scorpion Stretch _____ 57

Cobra Stretch _____ 59

Extended Puppy Stretch _____ 60

Reclined Twists _____ 62

Happy Baby Pose _____ 63

Bow Stretch _____ 64

Standing Half Forward Bend _____ 65

Plow Stretch _____ 67

Downward Facing Dog _____ 69

Plank Pose _____ 71

Upward facing dog _____ 72

Sphinx Stretch _____ 73

Reclined Pigeon Pose _____ 75

# Chapter 5: Morning Yoga Poses For The Legs
_____ **76**

Dolphin Pose _____ 76

Triangle Pose _____ 78

Half-moon Pose _____ 80

Upward extended feet pose _____ 82

Side Reclining Leg Lift Pose _____ 83

Extended Hand To Big Toe Pose _____ 85

Standing Splits _____ 87

Monkey Pose _____ 89

Hand Under Foot _____ 91

Waterfall Pose _____ 93

Chair Pose _____ 95

Heron Pose _____ 97

Dancer Pose _____ 99

Wide-legged Forward Pose _____ 101

## Chapter 6: Morning Yoga Stretches For The Hips _____ 103

Low Lunge _____ 104

Crescent Lunge _____ 106

| | |
|---|---|
| Lotus Pose | 107 |
| Eagle Pose | 108 |
| Lizard Pose | 110 |
| Twisted Monkey | 111 |
| Revolved Triangle Pose | 112 |
| Pigeon Pose | 114 |
| One-legged King Pigeon Pose | 116 |
| Horse Face Pose | 118 |
| Fire Log Pose | 120 |
| High Crescent Lunge | 122 |
| Cow Face Pose | 124 |
| Garland Pose | 126 |
| Crescent Moon With Back Bend | 127 |
| Horse Pose | 129 |
| Side Lunge | 131 |
| Wide Seated Forward Pose | 132 |

Three-legged pose ............................................. 134

Fire-fly Pose ...................................................... 135

## Chapter 7: Morning Yoga Stretches For The Chest _____ 138

Seated Chest Opener ........................................ 139

Supported Fish Pose ......................................... 141

Triceps Stretch ................................................... 143

Thread the Needle ............................................ 144

Noose Pose ......................................................... 146

Chest Opener With Blocks ............................... 148

King Cobra Pose ................................................ 150

Wild Thing .......................................................... 151

Half-frog Pose .................................................... 153

## Conclusion _____ 155

# Chapter 1: Understanding Yoga and Its Benefits

Let's start at the very beginning:

## What Is Yoga?

Yoga is a practice of the body and mind that includes meditation, body postures, and breathing techniques. At the most simplified level, morning yoga stretches are poses you do in the mornings to help your mind and body prepare for the day ahead.

The main idea behind yoga is to connect the mind, body, and soul; however, modern yoga focuses on strength, breathing, and exercise.

## The Origin Of Yoga and Its Evolution

Yoga dates back to 5000 years ago in Northern India. The Indians are said to have owned sacred texts known as the *Rig-Veda,* which contained mantras, songs, and rituals used by the priests and where the word *yoga* finds its first mention. Hindus recognized and continue to recognize yoga as one of the schools of philosophy and a vital part of Buddhism, along with its mediation practices.

In the pre-classical period, yoga did not involve posture and breathing practices; rather, it was a way of life. In the post-classical yoga period, yoga masters developed yoga practices meant to prolong life and restore the body and mind.

However, it was not until the late 1800s and early 1900s that these yoga masters began exploring the West and spreading their yoga works by writing books and establishing yoga centers.

In 1947, as the spread of yoga in the West continued, Indra Devi, a pioneering yoga teacher, opened a yoga studio in Hollywood. Since then, more Western and Indian teachers have become popular yoga pioneers with multiple followers, thus making yoga more popular globally.

## What Are The Health Benefits Of Yoga?

The practice of yoga utilizes techniques that focus on physical and mental well-being. When the participant is in a positive state of mind, healing and restoration happen faster than when the mind is in a negative state.

According to a study[2] done by the National Library of Medicine in 2011 to explore the therapeutic effects of yoga and its ability to increase the quality of life, the results showed the following benefits of yoga:

## *Improves pulmonary and cardiovascular function*

50 participants attending yoga classes were subjected to 75 minutes of daily yoga practice for 41 days. Pulmonary and cardiovascular tests were recorded before the yoga training began, then reassessed after 41 days.

According to the test results[3], there was a decrease in the participants' resting heart rate and blood pressure. Researchers concluded that yoga is beneficial in improving cardiovascular and pulmonary function.

---

[2] https://www.ncbi.nlm.nih.gov/pmc/articles/PMC3193654/#:~:text=Results%20from%20this%20study%20show,and%20enhance%20overall%20well%2Dbeing

[3] https://www.ncbi.nlm.nih.gov/pmc/articles/PMC5793005/

## *Enhances recovery from addiction*

Yoga can prove very helpful when the mind starts depending on alcohol and drugs. This may explain why recovery centers have used yoga to help affected individuals overcome withdrawal symptoms from the addiction and manage stress.

One main thing to note about addiction to certain substances is that it alters the brain. These alterations impact its function and structure because drugs and alcohol tend to fill the brain's nucleus accumbens and trigger high levels of dopamine, the neurotransmitter responsible for feelings of pleasure, motivation, and more.

When the dopamine levels are high, one feels encouraged to continue seeking the substances, making them feel as though they need them to survive or feel good.

A study[4] by the National Library of Medicine states that one core benefit of yoga is its ability to help return dopamine levels to normal. This is because the areas of the brain that help you be more attentive and mindful enlarge, which can

---

[4] https://www.ncbi.nlm.nih.gov/pmc/articles/PMC3525089/

help improve control over cravings and impulses, thus helping with maintaining sobriety.

Also, Yoga techniques like meditation involve mindfulness, which is repeated focus on the present moments while letting go of distracting thoughts and emotions. When sustained for long periods, one can control their mind.

## Improves sleep routines

Research[5] by the Journal of Ayurveda and Integrative Medicine in 2013 involved a group of 35 participants practicing yoga regularly for a long-term period of 5 years, and another group of yoga non-participants, with researchers then assessing the sleep patterns of both groups.

The results showed that those who practiced yoga had fewer sleep disturbances, took a short time to fall asleep, and showed a significant decrease in the use of sleeping pills. The researchers concluded that this effect was because yoga stretches tend to stretch and relax muscles, thus resulting in physical and mental exertion.

---

[5] https://www.ncbi.nlm.nih.gov/pmc/articles/PMC3667430/#:~:text=One%20possible%20reason%20explained%20for,disturbances%2C%20and%20better%20sleep%20efficiency.

### Better focus in the day

By doing morning yoga, you can declutter your mind through meditation and exercises that require balance, such as the one-leg balance, which requires focus. This will help force your brain to wake up and be ready to concentrate on the tasks ahead.

### Increases your energy and flexibility

When you stretch your body, your body muscles receive oxygen three times faster than when you are resting. The red blood cells are responsible for carrying the oxygen that the muscles need, and when one is active, the heart pumps and supplies the blood all over the body, including the muscles and energy cells. When your body gets the oxygen it needs, it becomes newly energized, making you feel fresher and more alert.

On the other hand, the more yoga stretches you do, the more you stretch your muscles which helps increase your flexibility and decrease the stiffness in the muscles.

## *Reduces your stress levels*

The human mind constantly races with thought after thought, many dwelling on past events or issues and possible future occurrences, which can be exhausting and stressful. Yoga utilizes techniques such as breathing and meditation that help clear the mind.

As you focus on breathing in and out or meditating, you get to manage those thoughts that lead to stress and clear your mind because you have to perform the poses with such concentration that stressful worries and thoughts are left out.

This helps you become more relaxed; therefore, you will not worry or become anxious about what lies ahead, like, a job meeting or being caught up in traffic on your way to work, because your stress levels will be down, and you can face the day with a more positive mind.

## *Your body becomes toned up*

Yoga stretches will give your body a better shape, with your back becoming stronger and arms being more defined, and you can even lose a few pounds. This is because you hold specific poses meant to tone specific muscles, and if you consistently repeat these poses several times during each session, it will tone up your body. Although it may take time before you notice the changes in your physical appearance, you need to be persistent; eventually, you will see the difference.

### *Set your day's intentions*

Your purpose for the day depends on what you personally aspire to achieve. For example, you may have the intention to be more confident, practice more gratitude, or be more kind towards yourself, especially your body.

During yoga, other thoughts in your mind begin to subside with the help of meditation and posture, thus bringing your intentions to the forefront of your mind. As your intentions become clear, you can draw inspiration from them as you strive to attain your goals. Whatever that aim is, it vitally shapes the rest of your day and helps you focus for hours ahead.

### *Helps get rid of the bodily fluids*

During the night, when we are asleep, our body muscles are resting, and bodily fluids start to build up between the muscles when they are immobile.

By stretching our bodies, we release the build-up of fluid between our muscles, contrary to when we do not stretch, leading to the build-up of the fluid in the muscles; thus, they become stiff and cause common body aches and pains.

## What about that coffee urge?

If you constantly feel the urge to take a cup of coffee to stay awake or focus on the day's tasks, you don't have to do that once you start doing yoga stretches. These stretches have a great way of relaxing, energizing, and stimulating the body and mind. You feel more awake or alert, and that need for coffee decreases with time.

## Can You Do Yoga From Home?

It is normal to imagine you have to walk or drive to a yoga studio to do your yoga stretches. But that is not so. You can do the stretches from the comfort of your home, and all you need is a workout mat or rug and some instructions to follow.

You now understand what yoga means and the benefits of starting your day with a morning yoga stretch routine.

## Morning Yoga Stretches

Before we discuss various morning yoga stretches and routines, let us learn how to breathe and let go during yoga.

# Chapter 2: Breathing and Letting Go During Yoga Stretches

As we all understand, breathing is vital to human existence, yet most of us only use a small portion of our lungs for breathing. The good thing is that rhythmic and deep breathing is a core pillar in yoga, which helps one get adequate oxygen through the entire body, thus ensuring it functions properly.

In addition to focusing on the breath, it is also important to let go of other thoughts and be in the moment. However, doing this is not easy and takes time to do so.

In this chapter, we will learn about yogic breathing patterns, how to let go, and the proper ways to breathe during various yoga poses.

## Yoga Breathing Patterns

- **Thoracic breathing:** This pattern involves breathing into the lungs upwards and outwards; in the process, the lungs expand as you draw in the air and drop when you breathe out.

*Morning Yoga Stretches*

- **Abdominal breathing:** Here, you breathe deep and long into the abdomen while concentrating on the expansion of the stomach as you breathe in and squeeze it in through the exhale.

- **Yogic breathing:** You take in one long and slow breath filling up the stomach, chest, shoulder, and neck areas. When exhaling, you start by releasing from the abdominal area, followed by the chest, shoulder, and, finally, the neck.

- **Clavicular breathing:** You breathe deep into your lungs until you feel the upper part of the lungs around the base of your neck expand and the shoulders move up. While breathing out, you slowly release from the chest, followed by the neck.

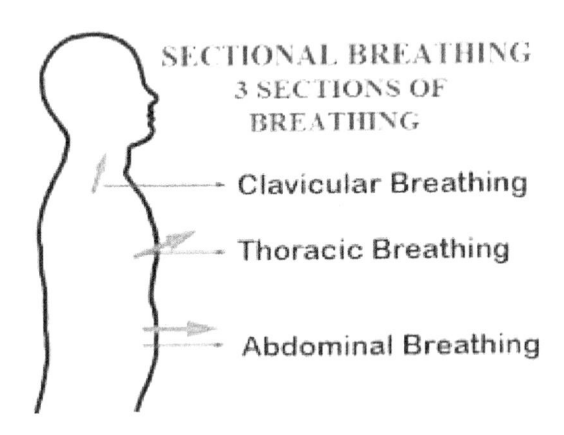

SECTIONAL BREATHING
3 SECTIONS OF
BREATHING

- Clavicular Breathing
- Thoracic Breathing
- Abdominal Breathing

# How to Breathe During Yoga

When doing yoga stretches, you mostly move your body from one position to another, with the poses coordinated with your breath.

Here are tips to help you breathe effectively during your yoga practices:

## *Up and down*

When you perform yoga stretches that require you to raise your arms overhead, raise your body upward, or lift your legs as you inhale.

When you move your body downwards, bring your arms down to your sides or lower your legs and exhale.

## *Preparation and movement*

Another way you can learn how to breathe is by focusing on your body movements. When in stillness and preparing to move your body, breathe in to fill your lungs with oxygen. In other words, you inhale to prepare your body for the movements.

*Morning Yoga Stretches*

When you move your body and engage your muscles through the yoga stretches, exhale. Breathing out braces your body during motion.

- When bending sideways, breathe out.

- When bending forward, exhale.

- When bending backward, exhale.

- When moving your body from the center position, exhale.

To ensure you breathe effectively during your stretches:

- **Sit or stand upright:** This way, you will ensure your spine is straight and supported by the back and abdominal muscles appropriately to allow for proper expansion and contraction of the ribcage. Arching your back restricts airflow in and out of the lungs because the chest collapses; thus, try to maintain a straight spine.

- **Take deep breaths:** When starting, take deep and slow breaths to fill your lungs and body with maximum oxygen and relax your body. Also, ensure that breathing in and out is smooth.

- **Maintain the rhythm:** Try to keep your breaths smooth even when doing a challenging yoga stretch or a simple one. Sometimes it is easy to forget how to breathe and find yourself catching a breath, especially when trying a more challenging stretch. That only means you are trying too hard, in a poor position, or using excessive force. If that is the case, slow down and deepen your breath.

If you are practicing yoga for the first time, do not hesitate if your breathing and movements do not match because this is normal; eventually, you will master both and reap the benefits.

## How To Let Go

Letting go means relaxing the entire body and letting your mind wander where it wants while you remain focused on your breath. If you have practiced yoga before, perhaps you have sat or lied on your mat with your mind filled with thoughts about finances, work, and relationships. This may have made you feel like you did not practice any yoga because your mind was full of distractions.

Well, here is where the beauty of the term letting go comes in because it helps you release the worries, stress, and other thoughts so that you receive the full relaxation and rejuvenation of the stretches.

So, how do you let go?

Here's are three practices that can help you do so easily, especially during your morning yoga practice:

## *Aparigraha:*

This is the practice of letting go of any attachment to feelings, patterns, habits, and even people that are either unnecessary, old, or anything standing in the way of our peace and freedom.

Think of a scenario where you are practicing yoga next to your friends or people you have invited to do the yoga stretches with you. Or when you are practicing alone and only thinking about being better than you already are. However, instead of focusing on what brought you there, perhaps being a better you, you focus on being better than the rest.

Aparigraha comes in here and allows us to focus on the practice without worrying about the material possessions, outcomes, or people we tend to rely on for happiness.

## *Replacing negative thoughts with positive thoughts*

With all the chaos in our lives, this idea is easier said than done, right? But everything requires practice, and the same goes for your thoughts and feelings.

The moment you notice yourself having thoughts of anger, disappointment, failure, or resentment, simply think of something positive, peaceful, and happy. Eventually, you will realize that this will be very beneficial during the day when you are worrying and planning, and replace the negative thoughts with positive ones.

## *Acceptance*

Sometimes accepting things as they are and riding along with them is better than pushing or fighting against them. Think of a surfer on a surfboard and how they ride on the wave easily. During yoga, instead of tensing up, breathe and accept your body's mental and physical responses that you cannot overcome immediately.

For example, accept that the bills, the toxic relationships, the everyday struggles, and responsibilities exist and will continue to exist. Nevertheless, you will not let them cloud or

*Morning Yoga Stretches*

burden your life. Instead, they are only part of the journey. By doing so, you help yourself thrive.

# Chapter 3: Tips To Get You Started With Your Morning Yoga Routine

We have seen all the amazing benefits of morning yoga stretches, but despite all that, you may feel like you do not have enough time for yoga practice, especially if you are a morning person.

Some people have to be up early for work; others are parents who have to prepare their kids for school. On the other hand, some people do not feel like they have enough energy to wake up early to work out, but it is not just a workout, is it?

Whatever your reason may be, the following tips will help you get started on your morning yoga routine and make it fun and rewarding enough for the brain to keep wanting to do it!

### *Prepare early in advance*

Preparing for something gets us ready for it; the same goes for morning yoga. The more effort you put into getting ready, the less likely you are to miss out on your yoga. So, prepare everything you need for your morning routine before you sleep the previous night. Have your space and equipment ready and roll out your exercise mat, so you do not have to waste time doing so in the morning.

Also, try eating a lighter meal at least three hours before bedtime because overeating too close to bedtime can interfere with digestion, thus affecting your sleep. In addition, ensure you get enough sleep, which is at least 7 hours, so you will be well rested in the morning.

If you have trouble falling asleep, try spending less time in front of your screen before bedtime and be more active during the day by incorporating some exercises into your day's schedule.

### *Think of the benefits*

If you do not feel constantly motivated to wake up and do your stretches, think of the rewards you will get from the routine—we discussed many in the previous chapter. Focus on getting through the day successfully instead of thinking about how you must get up early. Being physically and mentally healthy and improving your overall well-being should be your most important workout motivations.

## *Be realistic with your goals*

We all have an idea of what we want to achieve from the routine, but as much as the goals need to be clear, they should also be realistic. If you set goals far beyond you, you may end up overworking and straining yourself, thus giving up easily if you do not achieve them.

On the other hand, if your goals do not challenge you a bit, you may not feel challenged enough to want to continue because goals that are too easy and quick to achieve are boring. You can think of your first goal as completing five repetitions of a stretch without stopping. Then you can progress once you are comfortable and certain you do not struggle too much to complete your repetitions.

## *When you think of goals, think SMART:*

- **Specific:** A specific goal is clear and well-defined. For example, your goal might be to improve your flexibility through yoga.

- **Measurable:** The progress toward achieving your goals should be measured; for instance, you can pose for 2 minutes without pain.

- **Attainable:** Your goals should be possible to achieve. Goals such as losing weight need patience and taking one step at a time, so when losing 10 pounds in a month may seem possible, be real with your target.

- **Realistic:** they should be within reach. If you can hold your poses for 30 seconds to 1 minute, then setting goals to hold the stretches for more than two minutes is alright.

- **Timely:** The starting time and the target time should be clearly defined.

## *Be your own alarm*

Being able to wake up peacefully without the sound of the alarm stressing you out is a great way to start your morning yoga routine. Although it may take time and practice before you make it a habit to wake up at the same time every day without your alarm, it goes a long way to setting a natural rhythm for your body.

You simply have to be consistent and patient and wake up at the same morning hour every day, including the weekends; eventually, you will notice that you naturally wake up on your own.

## *Keep things simple*

We all do several things when we get up in the morning, like showering, brushing our teeth, searching through the wardrobe for what to wear, making breakfast, and answering emails while having breakfast. If you have to prepare for yoga, you have to cut the list of the things you do to only two or three: get up, shower, and practice.

## *Take a breath*

Most of us are guilty of grabbing our smartphones first thing in the morning when we wake up and checking the latest news feed on social media before we can even acknowledge being awake. But all that will only stimulate your stress and distract your mind from yoga.

Instead, when you wake up, take a deep breath to bring yourself to the present moment and check in with your feelings so you can adjust if needed. That sets the pace for your morning routine and reminds you to take more deep breaths during the day when the daily responsibilities or routines threaten to take your mind off your best intentions.

## *Hydrate*

Keeping your body hydrated is essential before and during your practice as it helps increase your energy levels for your morning routine. Start your day by drinking a glass of water before practice and during the stretches to replace the fluids you lose due to sweating. If you forget to take water, it may help to keep a water bottle nearby where you can see it; this way, you will remember to hydrate.

## *Snacks only!*

It is best not to eat before practice, as the fasted cardio theory states that: the body depends on stored carbohydrates and fats for energy during workouts which in turn leads to higher levels of fat loss.

However, if you are genuinely hungry or feel your blood sugar level is low, you can have light and easy-to-digest snacks like fruits or smoothies. The only thing you must ensure is not to eat anything not considered a light snack before practice.

## *Warm-ups*

Yoga stretches require you to challenge and stretch the muscles, and getting into the poses without warming up can be very dangerous since the body is more prone to injuries.

It is crucial to warm up before you start the stretches because they help heat up the body muscles and increase blood flow. The muscles and joints also loosen, thus reducing their stiffness and becoming more flexible, which is very important during workouts as it prevents injuries caused by stiff joints and muscles.

Besides, those who skip warm-ups may find it difficult to get into more challenging poses because they are not flexible enough to do so it is a good idea to learn a few basic poses that will help you get ready for your session.

However, you do not need to do the full repetitions of the yoga warm-up poses because you are just relieving the tension and getting into a yoga mindset.

With those tips, let us now dive into the yoga stretches!

# Chapter 3: Basic Yoga Warm-Up Stretches

Below are yoga warm-up stretches you can do before you engage in your morning yoga stretches routine:

## Warm-up 1: Child's Pose

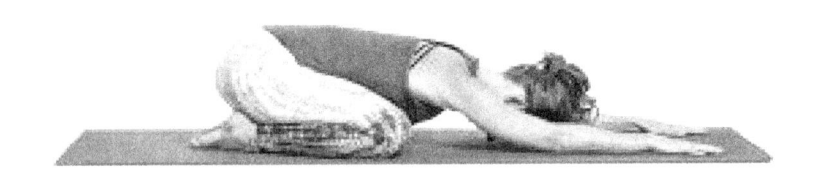

### Steps

- Start by going down on your knees in the center of your workout mat. Lower your body until your bottom sits on your heels, and your big toes touch each other.

- Part your knees until they are more than hip-width apart, then exhale as you slowly bend your upper body forward. Allow your torso to rest between the thighs such that your belly and chest almost touch the mat.

- Extend your arms in front of you with the palms facing down, and try to reach the top of the mat as far as possible.

- Hold this stretch for up to 3 minutes while concentrating on your breath. Let your thoughts go.

- Relax and return to the starting position.

*Morning Yoga Stretches*

## Warm-up 2: Hero pose

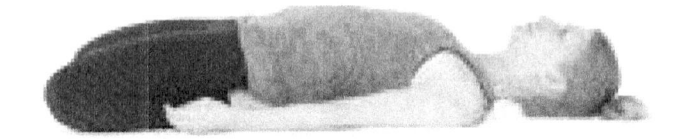

### *Steps*

- Go down to a kneeling position on your mat. Keep your feet apart and rest on the mat in the space between your feet with your heels on either side of your butt.

- Move your knees towards each other as far as you can until you feel a stretch in your thighs, ankles, and knees.

- With your hands on either side of your thighs, move them back toward your butt as you lean back, then bend at the elbows until your forearms rest on the mat.

- If you are comfortable on your forearms, you can continue to lean back further until your back rests on the floor and arms over your head or by your sides, but if your thighs, legs, and low back feel strained as you move your back toward the floor, simply stay on your forearms.

- Hold this pose and count up to ten breaths, then raise yourself back to the starting position. If you were down on your back, raise onto your forearms first, hands, and finally sit.

## Warm-up 3: Wide-leg Stretch

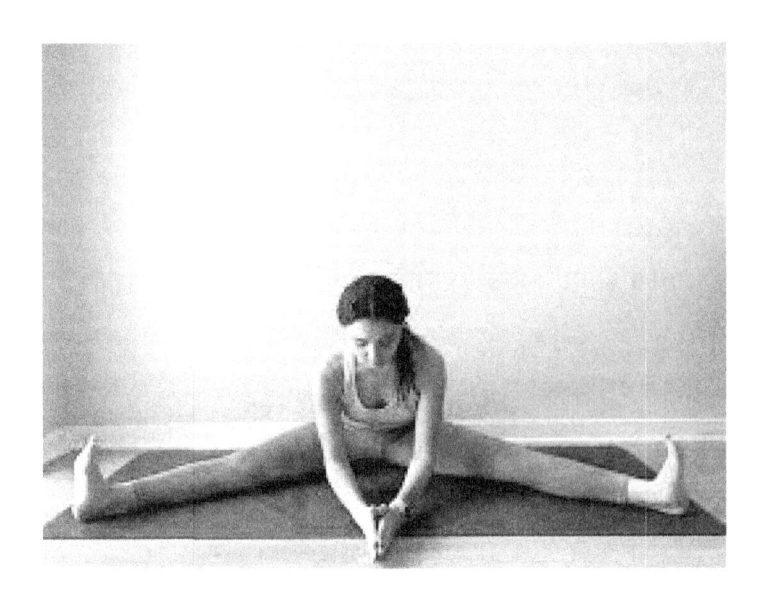

***Steps***

- Start by sitting at the center of your workout mat and extend your legs forward.

- Bring your legs wide apart as far as possible while keeping a straight back and flexing your ankles.

- Lean forward while moving your chest as close to one knee as you can, and rest both hands forward on the floor. Hold this position and count up to five breaths as you try to go deeper into the stretch on each exhale.

- Return to the starting position, then repeat the stretch on the other side.

*Morning Yoga Stretches*

## Warm-up 4: Cat and Cow

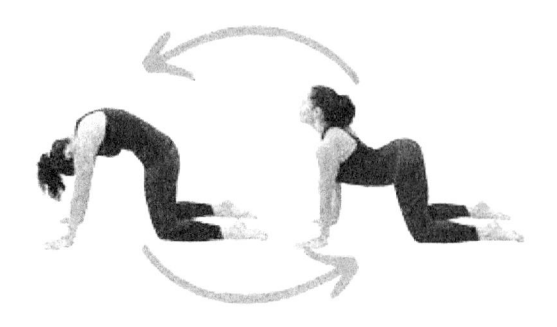

### *Steps*

- Start by going down on all fours until your legs and palms support your weight. Keep your knees hip-width apart and your hands shoulder-width apart. Your hands should face forward.

- Next, gently arch your back downwards while drawing in a deep breath while engaging your abdominals. You can face up for more tension on your back.

- Hold the position for a few breaths, curve your back upwards, and lower your head until you face down. Again, engage your abdominals.

- Repeat the stretch five times in each direction.

# Warm-up 5: Up and Down Hands Motion

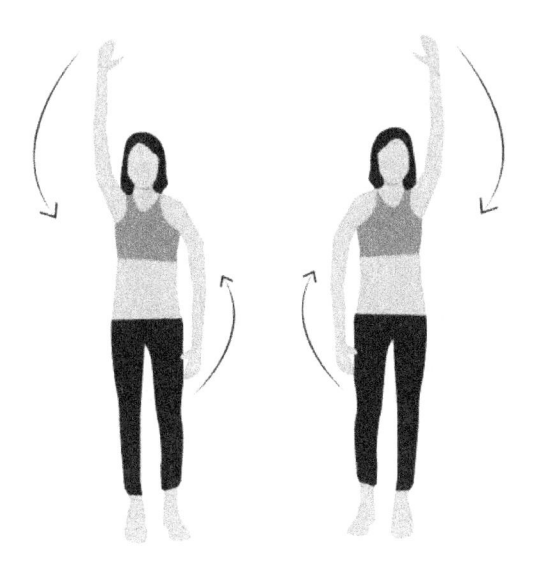

## *Steps*

- Stand upright and raise both hands at shoulder level.

- Next, inhale as you raise your right hand above the shoulder and lower your left hand at your side until both hands are straight.

- Exhale as you raise your left hand above your shoulder and lower the right hand until it is now at your side.

- Hold both positions for five to ten breaths.

_Morning Yoga Stretches_

## Warm-up 6: Neck Rotations

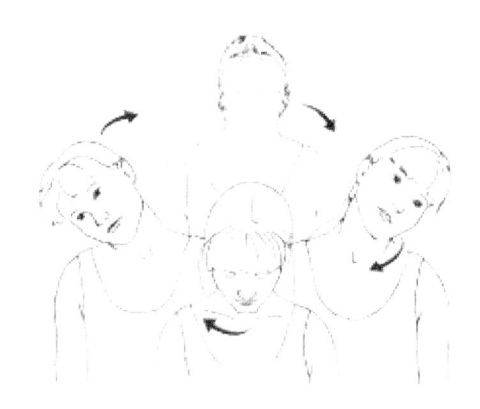

### Steps

- Stand upright with feet hip-width apart to ensure your head is in a neutral position.

- Next, rotate your head clockwise and count five breaths, then rotate in the anti-clockwise direction.

- Bring your head back to the neutral position as you breathe slowly and deeply and relax.

## Warm-up 7: Fish Pose

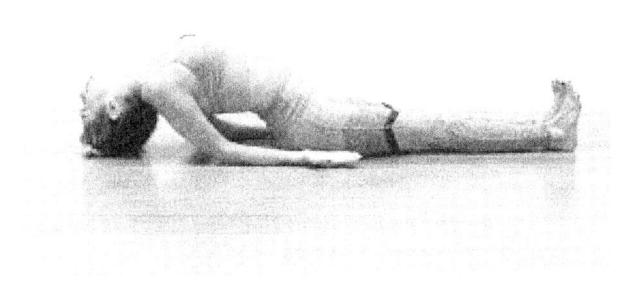

### *Steps*

- Place a mat on the ground then lie on your back and stretch your legs while placing your arms by the side and the palms facing down.

- Arch your upper back by lifting your chest while pressing your elbows and forearms into the floor for support. Raise your upper torso and shoulder blades off the floor while tilting your head back until the crown of your head touches the floor. Let your hands bear most of the weight by pressing them onto the floor, so your head bears less weight.

*Morning Yoga Stretches*

- Hold this position for five breaths, then release the pose by pressing into the elbows and forearms so you lift your head off the floor and lower your torso back to the floor.

## Warm-up 8: Tree Pose

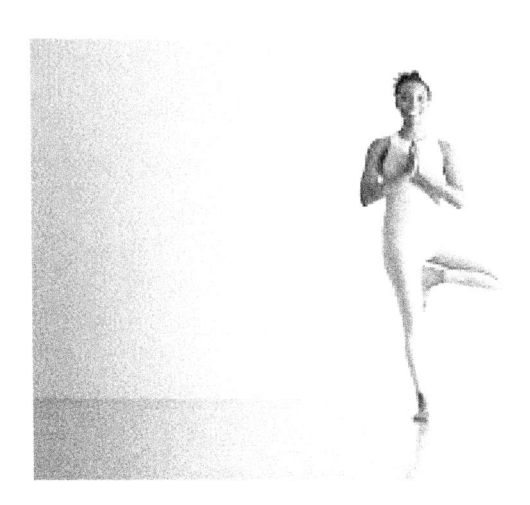

### *Steps*

- Stand upright with your feet close together and while you've placed your arms on the sides.

- Let your right foot bear your weight as you slowly and gently lift the left foot off the floor. Bring your left foot up until it aligns with your right thigh and your toes point down towards the floor. Keep your pelvis straight.

- Extend your arms upward and press the palms together to form a V.

*Morning Yoga Stretches*

- Hold this position for five breaths, then lower your leg back to the starting position.

- Repeat the stretch with the right foot. Focus your attention on your pose, breath, or any object in the room while performing the stretch.

## Warm-up 9: Easy Pose

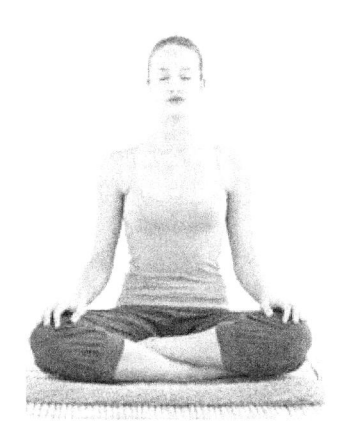

### *Steps*

- Start by sitting in the center of your workout mat.

- Cross your legs, then lean side to side and back and forth with your torso. Flex your shoulder blades downward to bring your shoulders away from your ears.

- Rest your hands on your laps with your palms facing up or down, then lengthen your spine as you inhale. Hold this position for five breaths, then release it to the original position.

## Warm-up 10: Staff Pose

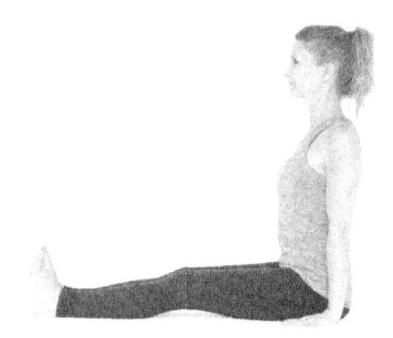

### *Steps*

- Sit in the center of your mat and extend your legs ahead of you with your toes facing up. Bring your toes together so they touch and so there is a small space between your heels.

- Bring your hands to your sides and stretch your arms.

- Flex your shoulder blades back and down your back, then bring them down toward each other.

- Slightly move your chin back and down while keeping the base of your neck smooth. Count five to ten breaths.

# Chapter 4: Morning Yoga Stretches For The Back

Here are the best yoga stretches to do in the morning to strengthen and soothe your back.

## Bridge Bends

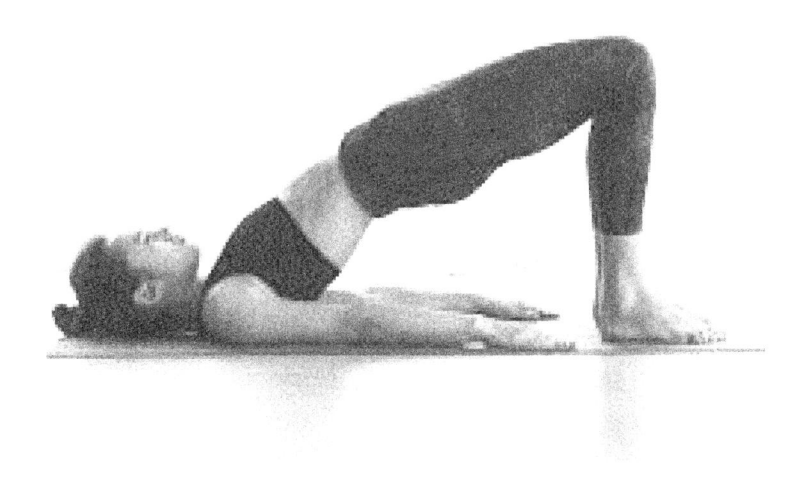

This stretch helps loosen up tight back muscles and joints.

*Morning Yoga Stretches*

## **Steps**

- Place a mat on the ground then lie on the back, making sure you put your arms on the sides. You can also interlace the arms under your back.

- Bend your knees at a right angle or until your feet are flat on the floor, then lift your hips up towards the ceiling.

- Lift your thighs up further until your shoulder tips are on the floor and the entire back is off the floor. You can place a block between your thighs to help perfect the form. Keep your arms straight.

- Count up to ten breaths, then release the pose.

# Seated Forward Yoga Bend

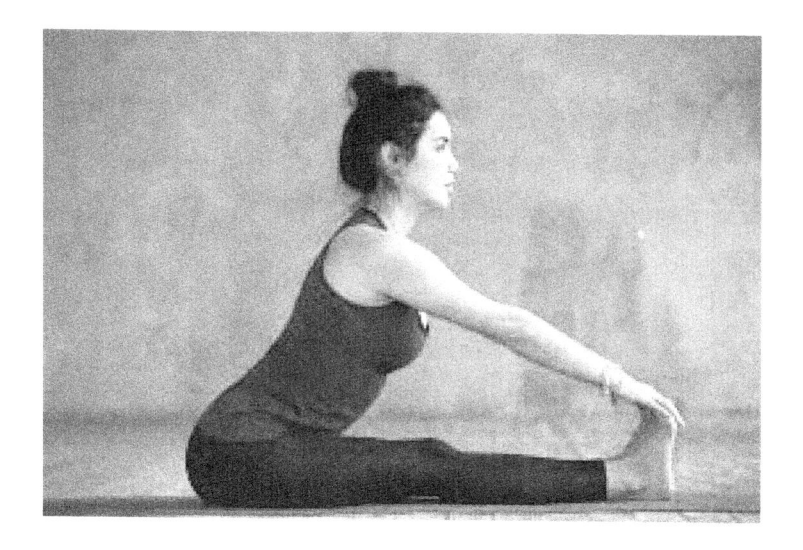

The seated forward bend gives your entire back a stretch from the neck to the heels.

## *Steps*

- Start by sitting on your mat with your legs outstretched in front of you.

- Lift your arms up over your head and extend them.

- Next, gently bend forward by hinging at the hips so you lower your torso towards the legs as far as possible. Keep your back straight.

*Morning Yoga Stretches*

- Extend your arms so you reach your hands toward your toes or heels. For a deeper stretch, flex your toes towards you as you press your heels out.

- Hold the position for ten breaths, then release the hold by gently moving your spine back to the starting position.

If you are flexible enough, you can try this variation of the stretch:

## Head-to-Knee Forward Bend

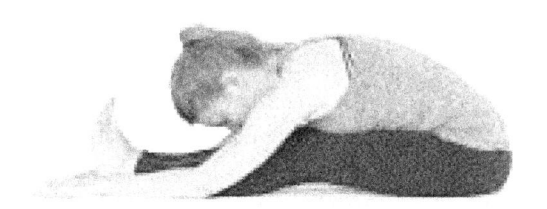

### *Steps*

- Start by sitting on a mat with your legs outstretched and lengthen your spine to keep your back straight.

- Hinge at the hips as you bend forward toward your legs from the belly, through your chest, and finally forehead.

- Slide your arms along the floor until they reach your feet, then let your fingers touch your toes. If you can't touch your toes, simply bend your elbows.

- For a deeper stretch, fold deeper into the pose until your nose touches your knees while maintaining a

*Morning Yoga Stretches*

straight back so your neck aligns with your spine. Keep your arms straight.

- Hold this pose for up to ten breaths, then release.

## Scorpion Stretch

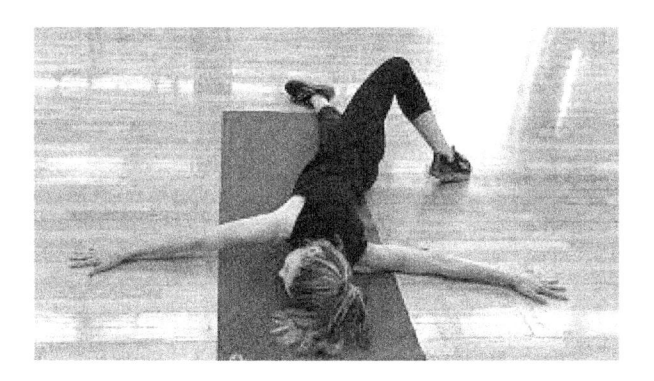

### *Steps*

- Lie on your mat facedown and extend your legs behind you with your arms outstretched at your sides until your body forms a T-like shape.

- Allow your chin to rest on the mat and look down to form a neutral spine from the neck to the tailbone. Keep your palms pressed lightly on the mat.

- Next, raise your right leg off the mat and bend at the knee to form a 90-degree angle, then bring your right foot across the other leg. Try to touch the floor outside the left leg with your right toes.

- Keep your chest and shoulders on the floor during the motion but only move the hips and lower back. You should feel a stretch in your lower back, right hip, and glutes.

- Hold this stretch for five breaths, then release and repeat on the opposite side.

## Cobra Stretch

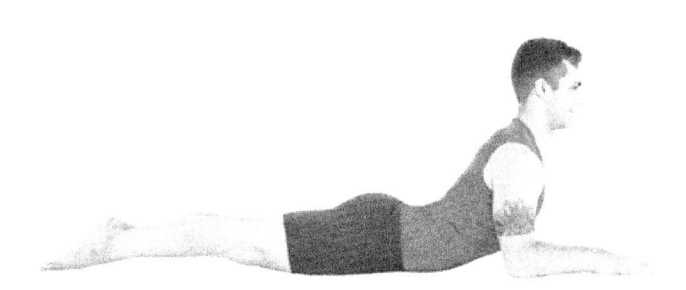

### *Steps*

- Start by lying on your belly with your legs extended behind you and hip-width apart.

- Bend the arms such that they take a 90-degree angle, so you rest on your forearms with the elbows positioned directly under the shoulders.

- Press the upper part of your feet into your mat, then flex your legs and rotate your inner thighs upward and outer thighs downward.

- Lift your chest off the floor and pull back against the resistance by pressing down into your forearms.

- Hold the stretch for ten breaths, then lower your chest to the mat while engaging your abdominals.

*Morning Yoga Stretches*

## Extended Puppy Stretch

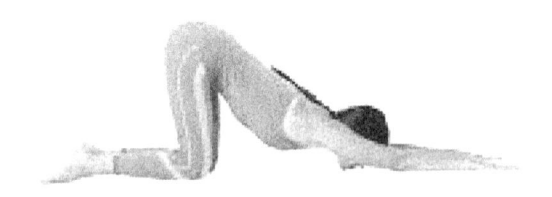

### *Steps*

- Start by coming down onto all fours so your hips are above your knees and shoulders above the wrists.

- Move your hands a few inches forward.

- Lower your forehead to the mat and relax your neck without dropping your elbows to the floor. Arch your back slightly and press your hands into the mat while extending your arms and pulling your hips backward to deepen the stretch.

- Hold the stretch and breathe deeply for 30 seconds-1 minute, then release.

## Reclined Twists

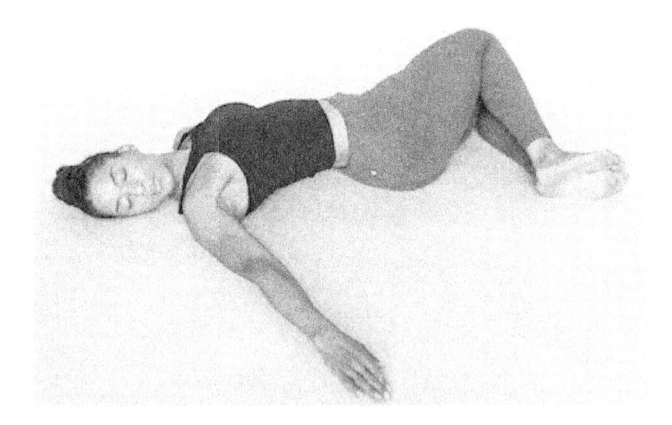

The stretch helps lengthen the spine, loosen the lower back muscles, and improve spine mobility.

### *Steps*

- Lie down on your back on a mat with your arms out to your sides, and bend your knees to have your feet flat on the floor.

- Lower your knees to your right until the thighs rest on the floor and face to your left.

- Count five deep breaths, then repeat the stretch on the other side.

# Happy Baby Pose

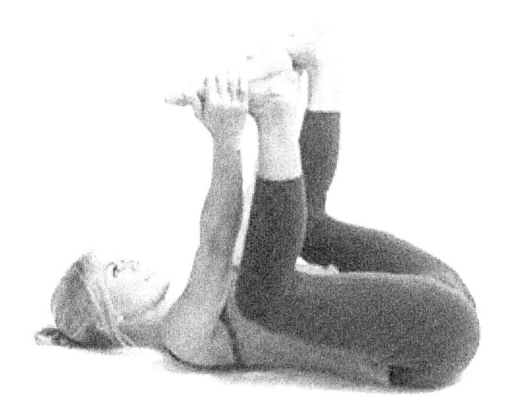

This yoga stretch helps loosen the lower back muscles.

## *Steps*

- Lie flat on your back on a mat with your legs relaxed.

- Lift your legs off the floor and bend your knees. Hold onto the feet and bring the knees toward your armpits.

- Relax in this position and count up to ten breaths, then release.

## Bow Stretch

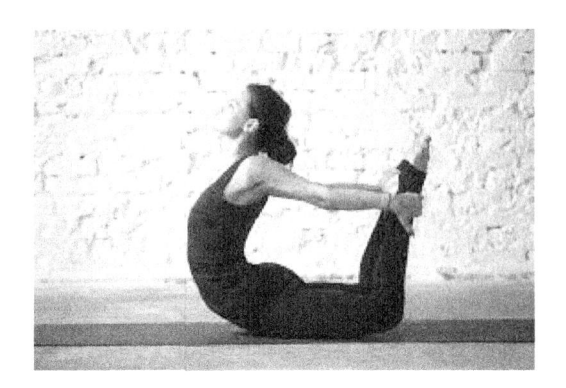

### Steps

- Start by laying facedown on your mat. Bend your knees and press the toes into the mat.

- Hold the outsides of your ankles using your hands while flexing your feet.

- Inhale as you raise your shoulders and rib cage up towards the ceiling. Exhale as you pull your tailbone toward your legs behind you.

- Lift your head and chest and face forward. Hold this stretch for 5-8 breaths, then release.

## Standing Half Forward Bend

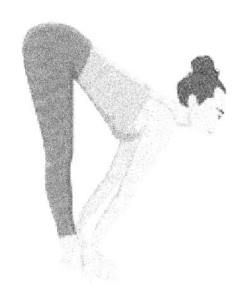

### *Steps*

- Stand upright with your feet together and bend forward.

- Keep your legs straight as you press your fingertips into the floor. If you can, press your palms beside your feet.

- Stretch your elbows as you bring your torso away from your thighs.

- Press down and back against the floor using your fingertips and lift your tailbone up and forward; you will slightly arch your back.

*Morning Yoga Stretches*

- Face forward and hold this position for up to ten breaths, then release.

## Plow Stretch

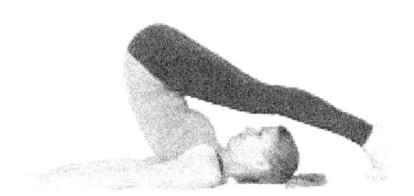

### *Steps*

- Place a mat on the ground then lie flat on the back, making sure to keep your palms facing down, arms on the side and your legs extended.

- Lift your hips and legs off the floor and up toward the ceiling while engaging your abdominal muscles. Continue lifting both and extend your legs until your torso is perpendicular to the floor.

- Gently and slowly lower your straight legs over your head until your toes touch the floor.

- With your arms still on the floor, extend them and interlace your fingers while pressing your upper arms firmly into the floor. Let your hips align over your shoulders.

- Hold the stretch for up to 20 breaths, then release. To come from the pose, use your hands to support your back, then gently return your back to the starting position.

## Downward Facing Dog

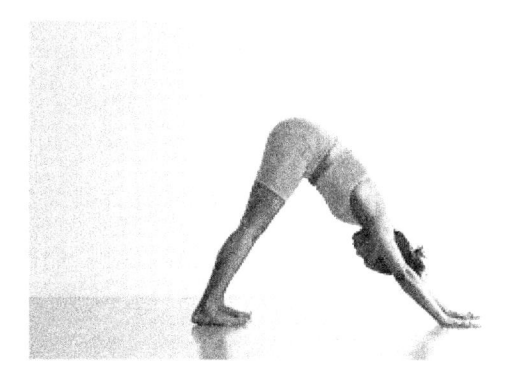

Apart from strengthening your back, the stretch also increases blood flow to your brain.

### *Steps*

- Go down on all fours until your hands are a few inches in front of your shoulders and knees underneath your hips.

- Curl your toes under your feet and press your palms into the floor as you lift your knees off the floor. Slightly bend and lift your knees off the floor as you also lift your heel off the floor.

- Lengthen your tailbone while lifting the sitting bones upwards. Bring your inner legs away from your ankles.

*Morning Yoga Stretches*

- Flex your heels downwards toward the floor while pushing your upper thighs backward. Begin gently straightening your knees.

- Press your fingertips into the floor as you extend your upper arms, then draw your shoulder blades toward your tailbone. Relax your head between your upper arms.

- Hold this pose for up to ten breaths, then release by first lowering your knees.

## Plank Pose

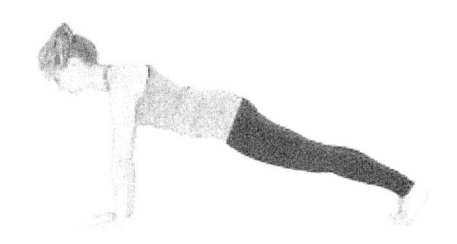

### *Steps*

- Go down on all fours until your hands are flat on the floor underneath your shoulders and knees underneath your hips. Keep your hands shoulder-distance apart.

- Straighten your legs behind you and lift your knees off the floor until your toes and hands support your weight. Your body should form a straight line.

- Keep your spine and neck neutrally positioned by gazing directly down and engaging your core.

- Hold the pose for up to ten breaths, then release.

*Morning Yoga Stretches*

## Upward facing dog

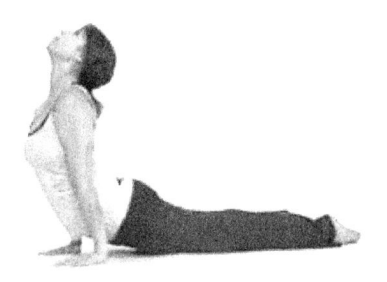

### *Steps*

- First, form a low plank by lowering your body halfway toward the floor. Keep your elbows near your sides.

- Lower your hips toward the floor and roll over your toes behind you until the top parts of your feet rest on the floor.

- Straighten your arms to lift your chest while squeezing in your core. Squeeze in your shoulder blades and look directly up to the ceiling.

- Hold the stretch for up to 20 breaths, then release.

## Sphinx Stretch

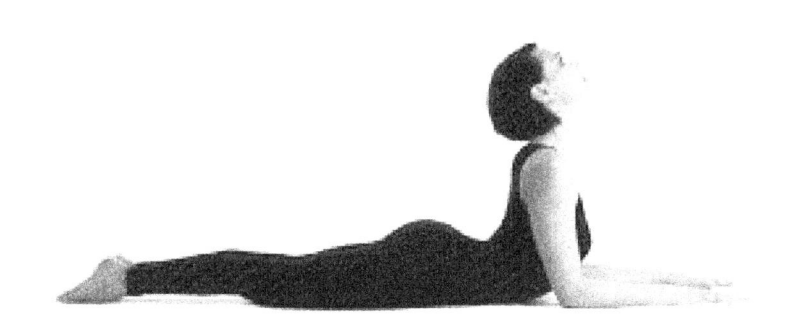

This stretch gives your lower back a nice curvature and strengthens the abdominal muscles to support the lower back.

### Steps

- Start by lying on your stomach and extend your legs behind you until they are straight.
- Bend your elbows until they are under your shoulders, and rest your forearms on the mat. Press your forearms into the floor and lift your chest off the mat.

*Morning Yoga Stretches*

- Lengthen your spine and relax your shoulders as you sit up until you feel a stretch in your lower back.

- Hold this pose for up to 20 breaths, then release.

## Reclined Pigeon Pose

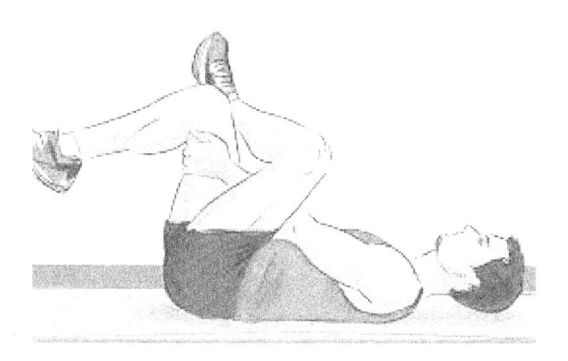

### *Steps*

- Lie on your back flat (on a mat) then bend your knees.

- Move your right foot across your left thigh while still bending your left knee.

- Grab the back of the left leg and then proceed to gently pull it toward the chest until you can feel a stretch.

- Hold this pose for up to 20 breaths, then release.

## Chapter 5: Morning Yoga Poses For The Legs

Let us now look at yoga stretches that will improve your legs' flexibility, balance, and strength.

### Dolphin Pose

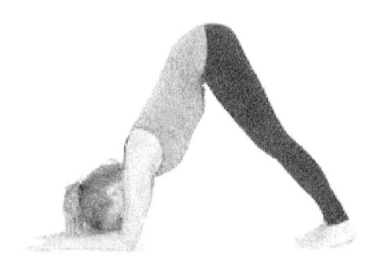

This pose stretches the calves and hamstrings.

### *Steps*

- Start by going down on all fours – (yound hands and knees) to have the wrists aligned with the shoulders and hips aligned with the knees. Your fingers should point directly in front of you.

- Bend at your elbows to form a 90-degrees angle from your shoulders. Your forearms should rest on the floor and parallel to each other. Let your weight be even on both forearms.

- Press your toes into the floor and gently lift your knees off the floor until your pelvis is toward the ceiling, then push your tailbone backward.

- Gently extend your legs behind you until they are straight, and keep your spine straight so your torso and legs form an 'A' shape. Ensure your feet and hands are not close to each other and that your back is not arched.

- Flex your shoulders inwards and toward your lower back, then relax your head between your upper arms. Focus your gaze between your legs.

- Hold this pose for 20 breaths, then release.

## Triangle Pose

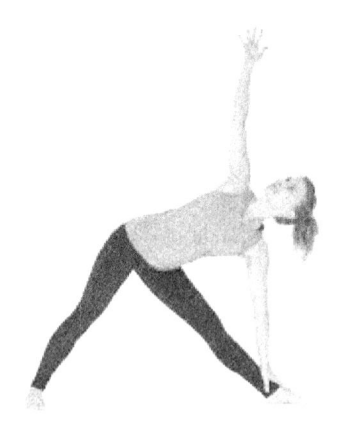

### *Steps*

- Stand upright with your feet a few inches apart and face the long side of your mat.

- Point your right toe toward the short edge of the mat and turn your left toe about 45 degrees in so you are stable. Your right thigh should align with the first two toes of the right foot.

- Lengthen your waist as you raise your arms until they are parallel to the floor.

- Lower your upper body to the right and extend it over the right leg while moving your hips towards the back.

- Lower your right arm towards the floor and place your hand on the floor, leg, or support if you can't reach the floor. Turn your ribs toward the ceiling.

- Lift your left arm toward the ceiling with your palm facing forward and your hand aligned with your shoulder.

- Lengthen your neck, keep it aligned with your spine, and gaze straight ahead or up at your fingertips.

- Hold this pose for 5-10 breaths, then release and repeat the stretch with the left leg forward.

## Half-moon Pose

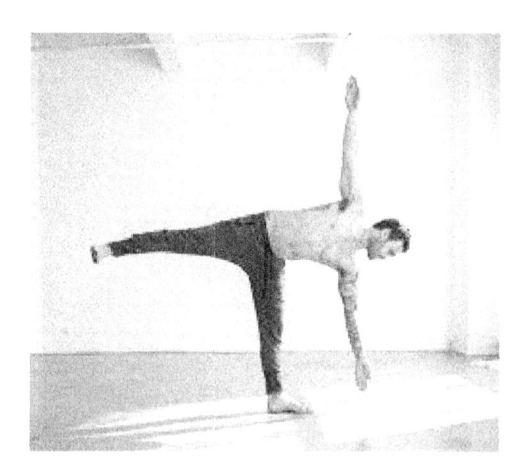

### Steps

- With your right leg forward from the triangle pose, gently bend your right knee and rest your left hand on your left hip.

- Lower your right hand toward the floor in front of your right foot and a few inches to the right of the foot until your fingertips slightly touch the floor.

- Raise your left foot off the floor gently while at the same time you straightening your right leg. Also, straighten your left leg.

- Move your left hip upward until the left hip point is on top of the right hip point.

- Continue lifting your left leg until it is parallel to the floor. Point your left toes to your left side.

- Once you gain your balance, lift your left arm up toward the ceiling until your left and right arms are perpendicular to the floor.

- Hold the pose for five breaths, then release and repeat the pose on the left side.

*Morning Yoga Stretches*

## Upward extended feet pose

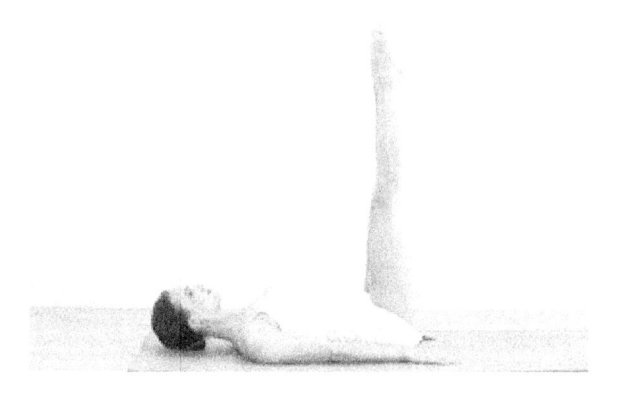

This stretch is great for releasing tension in the spine.

### *Steps*

- Start by lying flat on the back back on a mat and rest your hands by the sides with the palms facing up.

- Hinge your hips as you lift each leg until they are both perpendicular to the floor. Straighten your legs while engaging your core, and keep your lower back flat on the mat.

- Hold this pose for up to ten breaths, then release by lowering both legs back to the mat.

## Side Reclining Leg Lift Pose

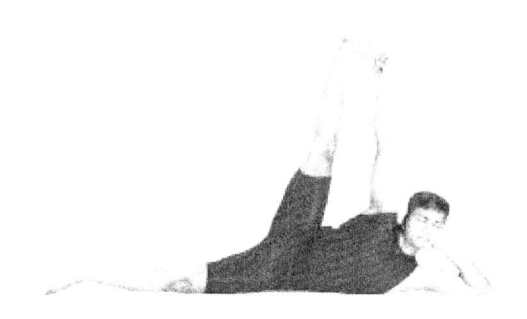

This stretch is great for lengthening and strengthening the backs of your legs.

### *Steps*

- Lie on your right side on the mat with your legs straight. Press your right heel into the mat while flexing the ankle, so you are stable.

- Extend your right arm along the floor, so your body forms a straight line from your fingertips to your heels. Bend at the elbow and use your palm to support your head. Stretch at the armpit.

- Lift your left leg up toward the ceiling, then bring your knee toward the torso by bending it. Rotate your leg,

*Morning Yoga Stretches*

    so the toes point towards your hand when you lift it. Grab the big toe with your left middle, index fingers, and thumb; you can also loop a strap around the heel and hold the end of the strap if holding using your fingers feels difficult.

- Extend the leg up while still holding it. Hold the pose for up to 15 breaths, then release and repeat with the right leg.

## Extended Hand To Big Toe Pose

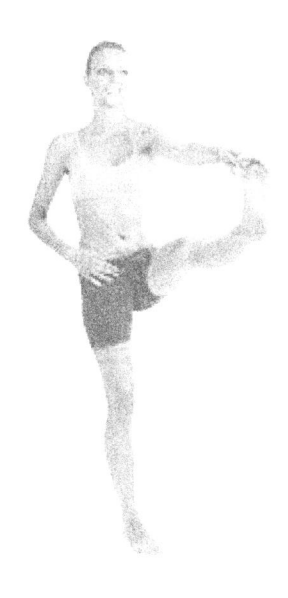

### *Steps*

- Stand with your feet hip-width apart and press your toes into the mat. Keep your back straight and your torso even on both sides.

- Keep the left leg firm on the floor, then bend at your right knee until you can hold the big toe with the index and middle fingers of the right hand.

- Push your right foot forward while keeping the hips even. If the right hip is higher than the left, lower it without bending your left leg.

*Morning Yoga Stretches*

- Hold this pose for about ten breaths or one minute, then release and repeat with the left leg.

## Standing Splits

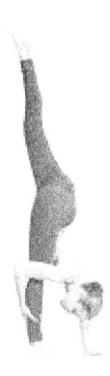

This stretch helps strengthen your ankles and knees.

### *Steps*

- Stand with your feet hip-width apart and bend forward from your waist. Place your palms flat on the mat with your fingers pointing in front of you.

- Balance your weight evenly on your fingertips until your back is straight.

- Lift your right leg behind you and point your toes back.

- Grab your left ankle with your left hand as you support yourself with the fingertips of your right hand. Lower your head toward the floor until the crown of your head points downwards.

- Continue to lift your right leg as high as you can as you draw your left hip in toward the middle until you press your inner thighs together.

- Hold this pose for a few breaths, then release and repeat with the left leg.

# Monkey Pose

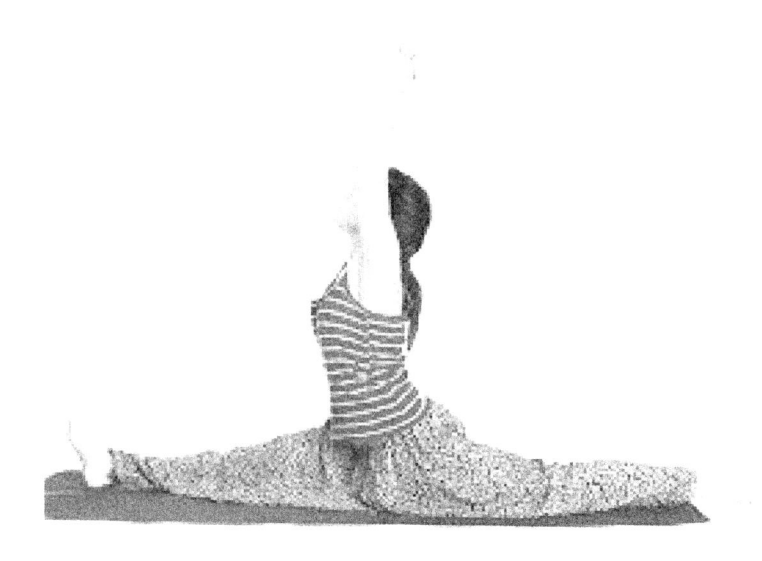

## *Steps*

- Start by descending on your knees with your thighs a few inches apart and perpendicular to the floor.

- Lower your hands in front of your knees until your fingertips touch the floor.

- Move your right leg forward and straighten it while keeping your heel on the floor.

- Continue to move your right foot forward while simultaneously extending the left foot behind you.

*Morning Yoga Stretches*

Keep your gaze forward as you extend your arms above your head and press your palms together.

- Hold the pose for up to ten breaths, then repeat on the other side. When you want to return to your starting position, bend your right knee, come onto the knee, and then bring your leg back towards your body.

# Hand Under Foot

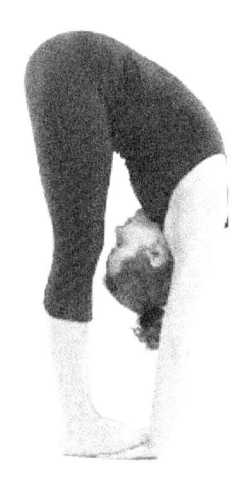

## *Steps*

- Stand on your mat with your feet close together and bend forward from your hips. Lengthen your torso and bend your knees as you bring your hands to the floor. Point the crown of your head toward the floor.

- Tilt your hands until your palms face up toward the ceiling and tuck them under your feet; your toes should touch your wrist joints. Let your weight balance evenly in your hands and wrists.

- Lengthen the back of your neck and shift your elbows out to your sides and forward.

*Morning Yoga Stretches*

- Hold the pose for up to ten breaths, then come out of the pose by bringing your hands from underneath your feet and back to the starting position.

# Waterfall Pose

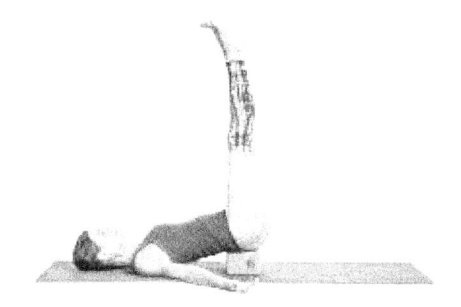

This stretch helps relieve any swelling in the legs and feet and is great for easing sciatica or varicose veins pain.

## *Steps*

- Lie flat on your back on a mat with your feet flat on the floor until your knees face the ceiling, with your arms relaxed by your sides.

- Press your feet into the mat as you lift your hips toward the ceiling, and place a block or pillow under your sacrum to support your pelvis.

- Next, bring each knee in toward your chest and extend each leg straight up toward the ceiling.

*Morning Yoga Stretches*

- Relax in this position for ten or more breaths, then return your legs to the starting position.

# Chair Pose

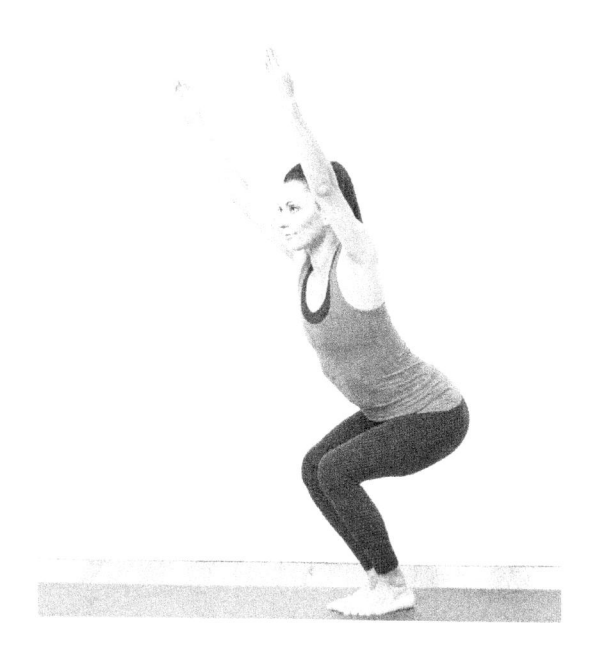

## *Steps*

- Stand upright with your feet together and lift your arms over your head, palms facing each other or pressed together.

- Bend your knees at 90 degrees angle so they are slightly in front of your feet, and your torso forms a right angle with the upper thighs. Your inner thighs should be parallel to each other.

*Morning Yoga Stretches*

- Squeeze your shoulder blades in and lower your tailbone toward the floor to lengthen your back.

- Hold this pose for up to 10 breaths or 30 seconds, then come back to the starting position.

# Heron Pose

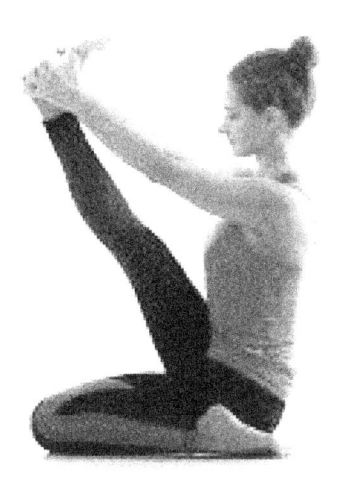

## *Steps*

- Sit upright on your mat with your legs straight in front of you.

- Bring your left leg back and bend at your knee until your left foot is outside your hip and straight, pointing behind you.

- Bend your right knee and bring the right foot closer to the hip joint. Hold the foot with both hands, lift it off the floor, and then extend the right leg as high as possible. Do not arch your back during the motion.

*Morning Yoga Stretches*

- Hold this pose for a few breaths, then release and repeat on the left side.

## Dancer Pose

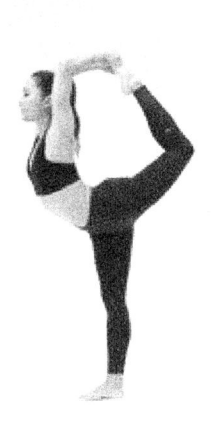

### *Steps*

- Stand upright with your feet together and hands by your sides.

- Lift your left leg off the floor and grasp your kneecap with both hands, then bring your knee in toward your chest while pressing down your right foot.

- Lower the bent knee down so the kneecap points toward the floor and is in line with the right leg.

- Bring the lifted left foot up behind you as you slightly bend forward. Grasp the foot with your left hand.

*Morning Yoga Stretches*

- Bring your right arm across your body to hold the left foot.

- Bring your left elbow out to your sides and turn your palm up so you hold the outer edge of your foot.

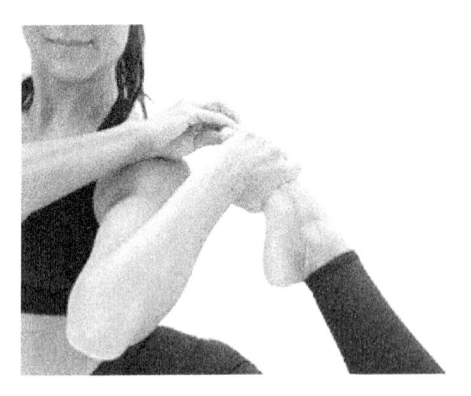

- Release your right hand from the grip and turn your chest forward as you lift your elbow up toward the ceiling.

- Bring your right arm up behind you and grasp the left foot.

- Hold this pose for a few breaths, then release and repeat with the right leg.

## Wide-legged Forward Pose

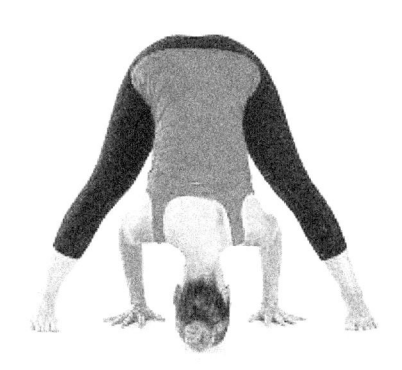

### *Steps*

- Stand on your mat and bring your feet wide apart and as parallel as possible. Place your hands on your hips.

- Lengthen your torso and bend forward from your hips without arching your back. Lower your body until your palms are flat on the floor with hands shoulder-width apart. Stretch your torso forward.

- Continue bending deeper until your crown points toward the floor while engaging your leg and thigh muscles. Lengthen your spine.

*Morning Yoga Stretches*

- Hold this pose for a few breaths, then slowly lift up to the starting position.

- Chapter 6: Morning Yoga Stretches For The Hips

If you sit for long periods at work, your hips need stretching too to prevent tight hips, which is a common issue in people who lead a sedentary lifestyle.

Here are a few yoga stretches you can commit to doing to keep your hips feeling good!

_Morning Yoga Stretches_

## Low Lunge

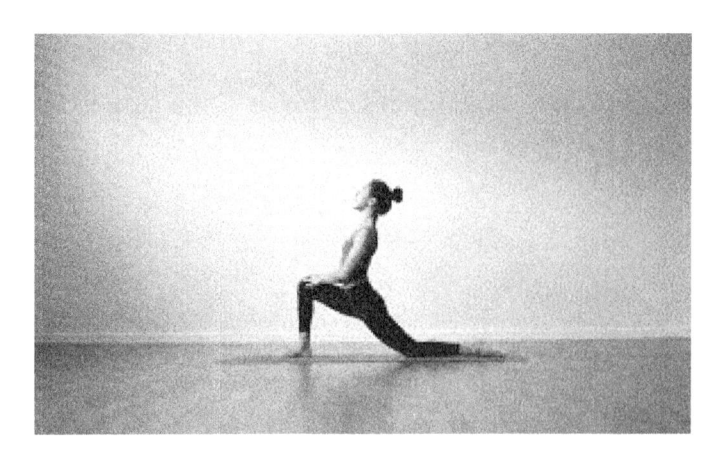

### Steps

- Start in the downward-facing dog pose and move your right foot forward between your hands.

- Go down onto your left knee until the top of the left foot rests on the ground.

- Keep the right knee directly over the right ankle so it does not move forward toward the toes or outward. The stretch you feel in your thigh and groin area should be comfortable. You can move your foot an inch forward for a deeper stretch.

- Come onto your fingertips on the floor on either side of your hips, or relax your hands on the front knee. Let your hips bear the weight of your body and stretch your tailbone down toward the floor.

- Hold the pose for 5-10 breaths, then repeat with the left knee bent and right leg straight behind you.

## Crescent Lunge

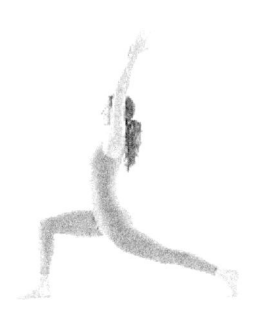

### *Steps*

- From the low lunge pose, straighten the leg behind you until you come onto the toes of the back foot.

- Lift your hands above your head with your palms facing each other and press them together. Gaze slightly above you.

- Hold this pose for ten breaths or 30 seconds, then release and repeat on the other side.

# Lotus Pose

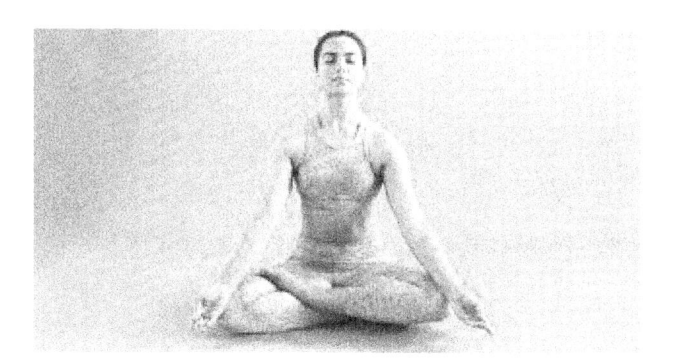

## *Steps*

- Sit upright on your mat with your legs straight in front of you and arms relaxed by your sides.

- Bend your right knee and bring it toward your chest. Grab the right ankle and pull it toward the hip line.

- Bend your left knee and bring it toward your chest. Rest the ankle in the hipline.

- Relax both hands on your knees with palms facing up.

- For a deeper stretch, place your hands beside your hips, press the palms into the floor, then lift your legs and buttocks off the floor.

- Hold this pose for up to ten breaths, then release.

## Eagle Pose

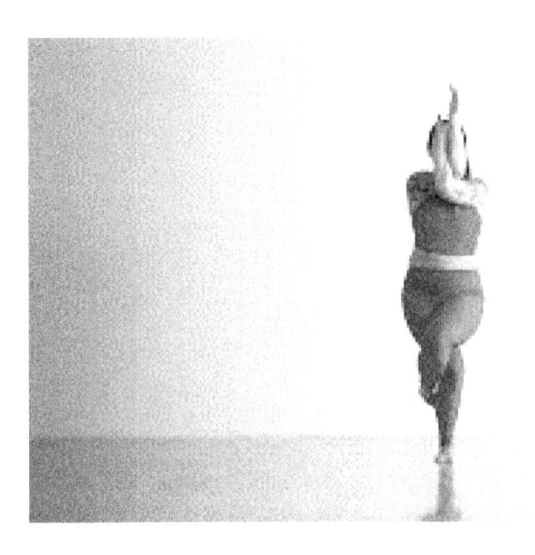

### *Steps*

- Stand with your feet slightly apart and place your hands on your hips.

- Use your hands to press your pelvis down toward the floor, so you lengthen your spine and feel the crown of your head lift up.

- Bend at your knees and lift your right foot, so you wrap your right thigh over your left thigh. Keep your left knee facing forward.

- Bring both arms forward and wrap your right arm over your left arm, so you cross the right elbow over the left upper arm. Move your left hand toward your face, cross the forearms and bring the palms together. Lift your elbow to shoulder level.

Hold this pose for five deep breaths, then release.

*Morning Yoga Stretches*

## Lizard Pose

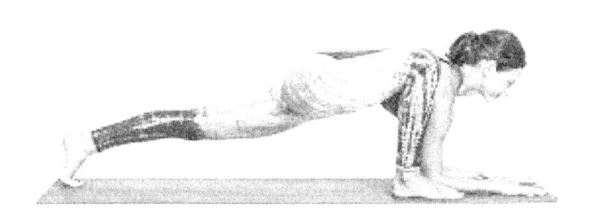

### *Steps*

- From the low lunge pose, move your right foot an inch out to your right side with your hands on the floor inside your front knee.

- Lift your left knee off the floor and come up onto your hands or your forearms for a deeper stretch.

- Hold this pose for a few deep breaths, then release.

# Twisted Monkey

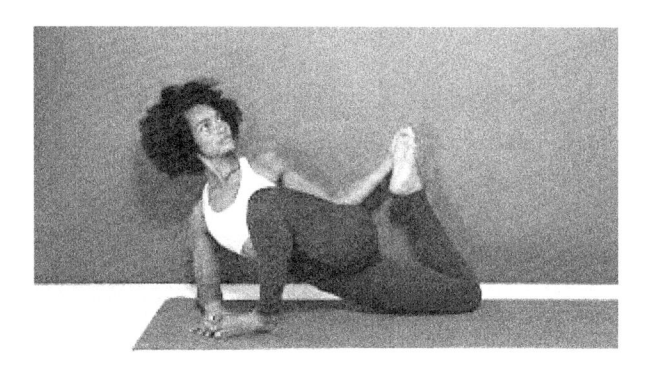

## *Steps*

- From the lizard pose, move the back knee back to the floor and bend your knee so the toes point up.

- Stretch your opposite arm and hold your outer foot. Rotate your spine so your chest faces up toward the ceiling.

- Hold this pose for a few breaths or ten seconds, then release.

*Morning Yoga Stretches*

## Revolved Triangle Pose

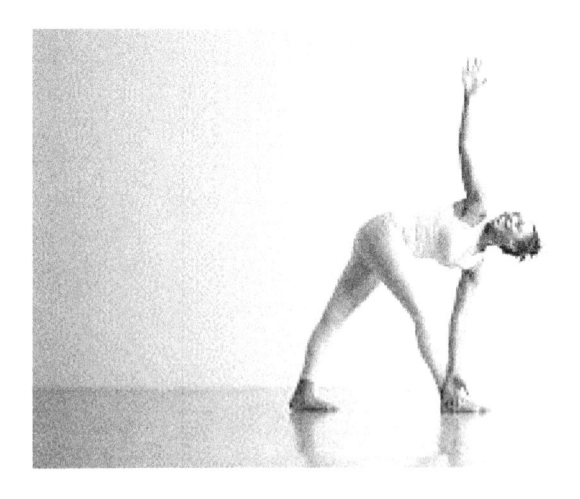

### *Steps*

- Stand on your mat with your feet together. Step your right foot about four feet forward and raise both arms to your sides until they are parallel to the floor. Open your shoulder blades wide with the palms facing down.

- Tilt your left foot slightly in so it faces your other foot, and turn your right foot out to 90 degrees. Your left heel should align with your right heel, and your right kneecap should align with the center of the right ankle.

- Stretch your torso to the right and bend from your hip joint while pressing your left heel into the floor.

- Next, tilt your torso toward the left while lengthening both sides of your torso. Bring your hip slightly forward and lower your tailbone toward the heel behind you.

- Bring your right hand to rest on your ankle or the mat outside your right foot. Extend your left arm up toward the ceiling until it aligns with your shoulder tops, and gaze toward the left.

- Hold this pose for 10 deep breaths or 30 seconds, then bring your body back to the starting position.

## Pigeon Pose

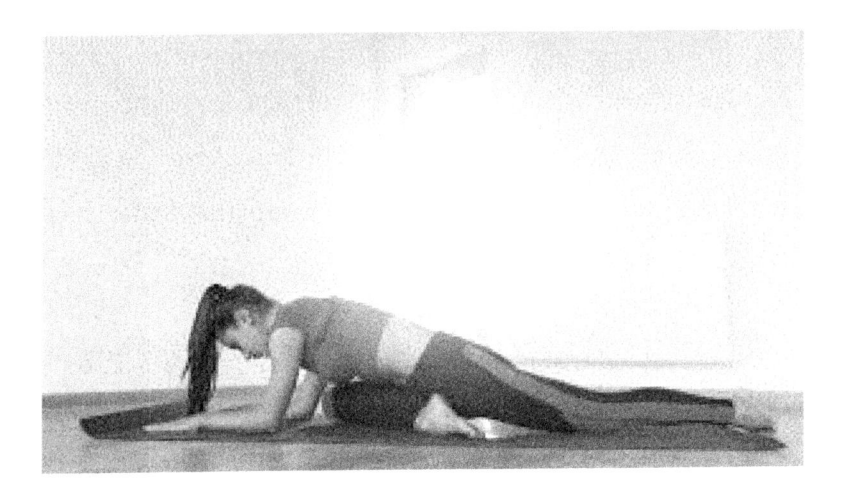

### Steps

- Come down on all fours on your mat. Curl your right leg at the knee and bring it forward so the kneecap is behind your wrist or to the inner or outer edge of the wrist—your right ankle should be in front of your left hip.

- You should feel a comfortable stretch in your outer hips and no pain or discomfort in your knee.

- Extend your left leg back behind you so your toes point down and your heel points up toward the ceiling.

- Bring both legs toward each other while keeping your hips level, then lengthen your spine as you come up onto your fingertips. Bring your hands forward and bend from your hips as you lower your upper body toward the floor.

- Let your forearms rest on the mat.

- Hold this pose for a few deep breaths, then bring your body back to the starting position and repeat on the other side.

## One-legged King Pigeon Pose

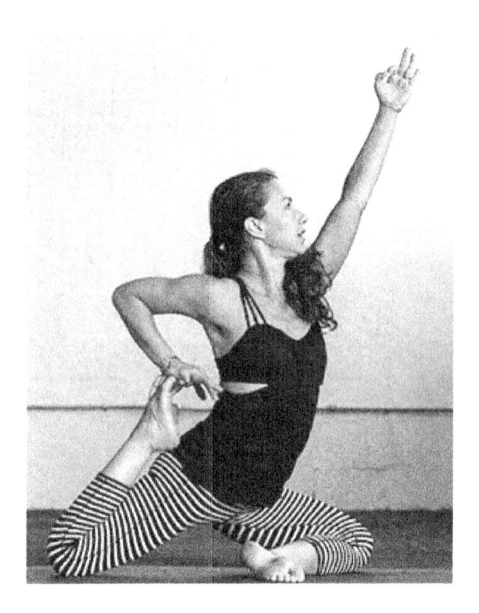

### Steps

- From the pigeon pose, bend the knee behind you until you reach for the ankle with the same-side hand. You should feel a stretch in your thigh.

- If you can, reach for the ankle with both hands while engaging your abdominal muscles.

- Reach the opposite arm up and forward to deepen the stretch.

- Hold the pose for five deep breaths, then release and repeat on the other side.

*Morning Yoga Stretches*

# Horse Face Pose

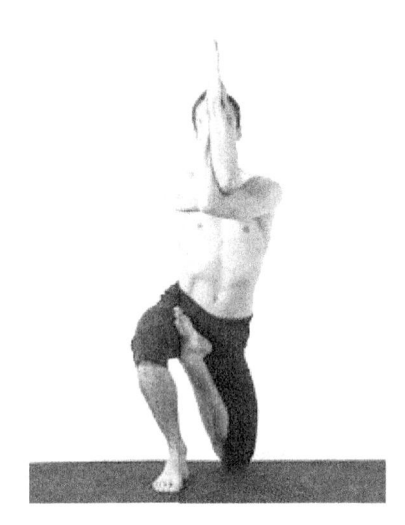

## *Steps*

- Sit on a mat with your back straight and hands by your sides, and bring your left foot over the right thigh near the hip line.

- Lift your torso off the floor and let your left knee touch the floor.

- Slide your right foot forward so your right heel is close to your left heel. Your right thigh should be parallel to the floor.

## Morning Yoga Stretches

- Raise your hands so they are level with your chest, and keep your back straight. Bend at the elbows, then cross them until the right elbow is over the left.

- Wrap your forearms and press your palms against each other.

- Hold this pose for up to 1 minute, then release and repeat on the other side.

*Morning Yoga Stretches*

# Fire Log Pose

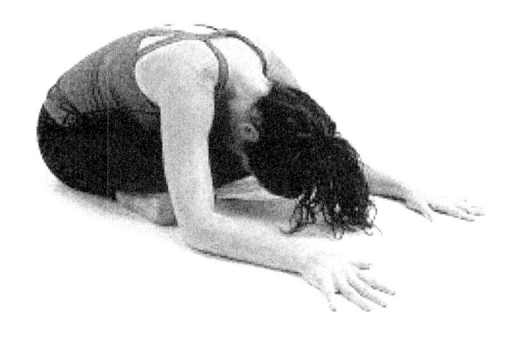

## *Steps*

- Sit upright on your mat with your knees bent and feet flat on the floor. Move your shoulders up and squeeze in your shoulder blades.

- Bring your left foot under your right leg until it is outside your right hip. Place your right leg on top of your left leg until the right ankle is outside the left knee.

- Lengthen your front torso as you bring your upper body forward from your hips. Bring your hands to the floor in front of your legs until your forearms rest on the floor.

- Continue folding deeper forward as you exhale.

- Hold this pose for a few deep breaths or 1 minute, then release.

*Morning Yoga Stretches*

## High Crescent Lunge

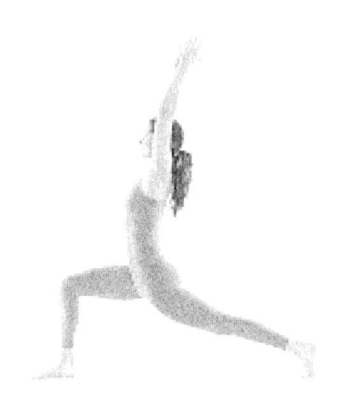

### *Steps*

- Stand on your mat and make one big step forward with your right foot until the distance between your feet is almost the length of the mat.

- Bend your right knee and extend your left leg behind you so it is straight and the heel is off the floor. Your right thigh should be parallel to the floor.

- Bring your hips forward until they are even.

- Lift both arms up and extend them over your head while pressing your front foot and toes into the mat until you feel a stretch in your hips.

- Hold the stretch for 5-10 breaths, then release and repeat on the other side.

## Cow Face Pose

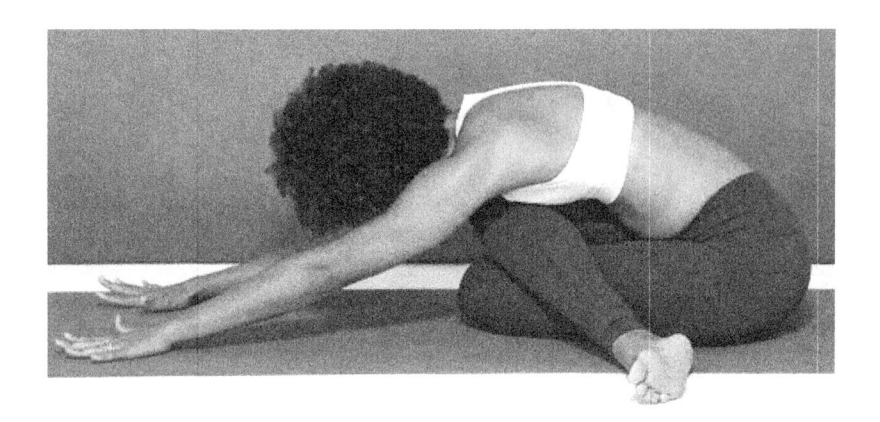

### Steps

- Go down on all fours, then cross one knee atop the other, so they are aligned.

- Move your knees farther from each other until your hips sit between your feet. Make sure one hip is not higher than the other, and if so, sit on a block to have them even.

- Sit upright, but if you want to deepen the stretch, bend forward from your hips until your torso touches your thighs and extend your arms in front of you, so your palms are flat into the mat.

- Hold the pose for at least five deep breaths, then return to the starting position. Repeat the pose on the other side.

## Garland Pose

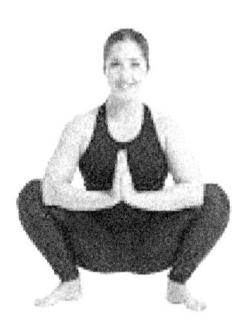

### Steps

- Start from a squatting position with your feet a few inches more than shoulder-width apart and flat on the mat. Lengthen your torso until it is upright and facing up.

- Bring your arms to your chest and press your palms together into a prayer position. Point out your elbows to your sides.

- Widen your knees more using the elbows.

- Hold the pose for five deep breaths.

## Crescent Moon With Back Bend

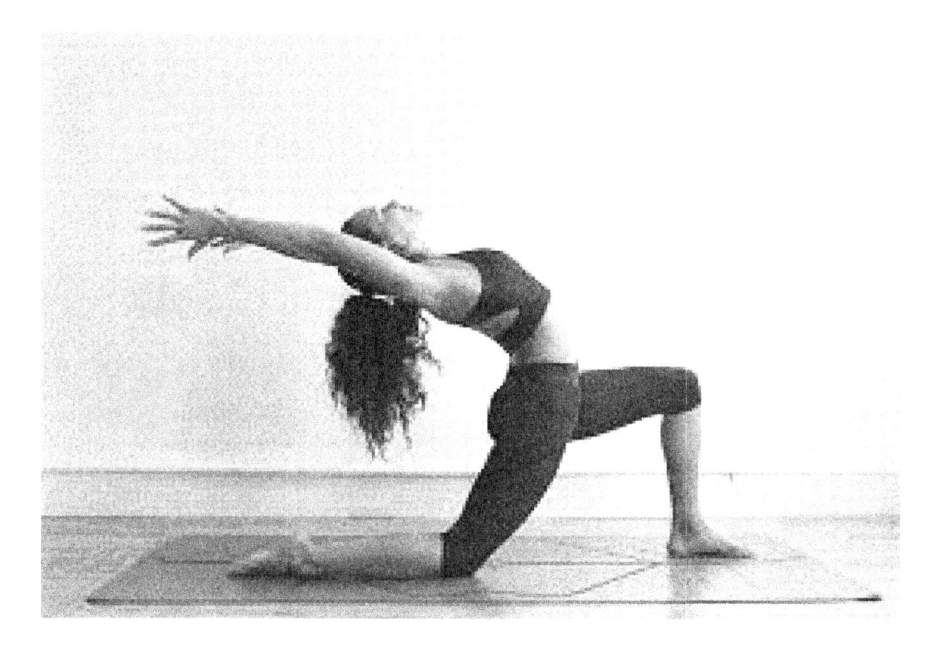

### *Steps*

- From the crescent lunge, bring both arms out to your sides.

- Gently press your hips forward and open your chest. Gaze up toward the ceiling and extend your arms above your head.

*Morning Yoga Stretches*

- Squeeze your shoulder blades toward each other and bring your torso up.

## Horse Pose

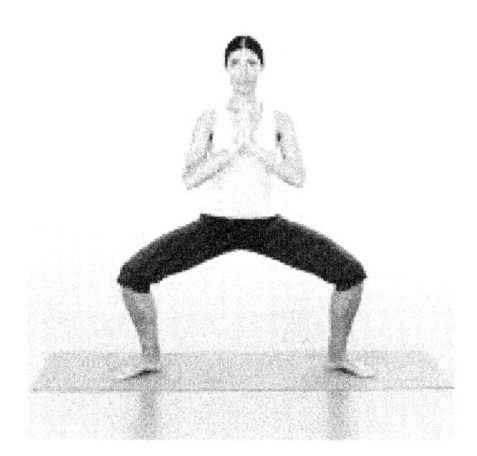

### *Steps*

- Stand upright with your legs wider than hip-distance apart and toes pointing out slightly.

- Bend your knees until your thighs are almost parallel to the floor, and lower your hips toward the floor as if you are about to sit.

- Bring your arms in front of your chest and press your palms together.

- Hold the pose for up to ten breaths,

*Morning Yoga Stretches*

- Try coming up onto your forefoot for a deeper stretch and balance your weight evenly.

# Side Lunge

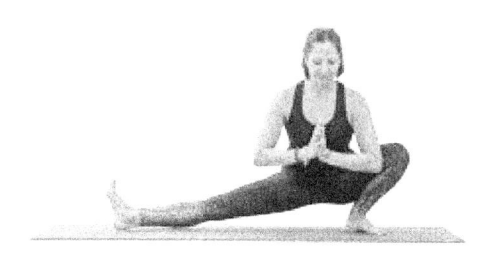

## Steps

- Stand with your feet together. Take one big step with your right foot to your side. Keep your feet flat on the floor and your toes pointing in the same direction. Bring your arms in front of you and press your palms together into a prayer position.

- Step your left foot outward while bending the left knee and keep the right leg straight. Come into your right heel and left foot. Keep your body lifted.

- Stay in this pose for a few deep breaths, then release and repeat on the other side.

*Morning Yoga Stretches*

## Wide Seated Forward Pose

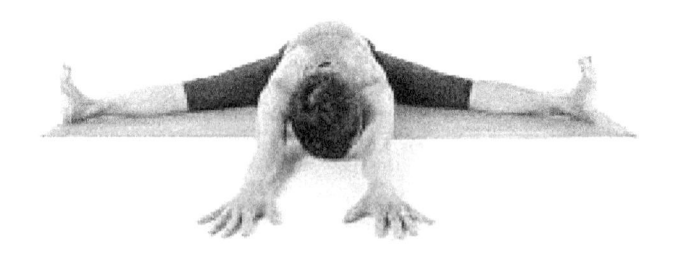

### *Steps*

- Sit on your mat and stretch your legs to your sides as wide as possible.

- Slightly bend your knees and point your toes up.

- Lengthen your spine and bend forward toward the floor from your hips. Extend your hands along the floor in front of you with palms facing down until your torso touches the floor between your legs.

- Rest the forehead on the floor and keep your back straight.

- Hold the pose for a few breaths, then return to the sitting position.

## Three-legged pose

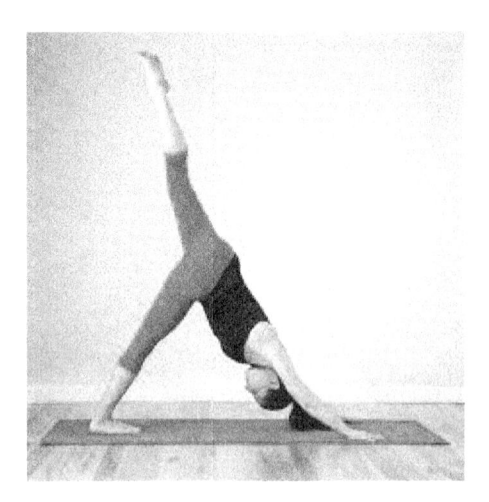

### Steps

- Begin in the downward-facing dog pose. Lift your right leg off the mat up toward the ceiling. Balance your weight evenly on both palms and left foot, and keep your shoulders level.

- Keep your head between your upper arms and right leg straight.

- Hold this pose for a few deep breaths, then come out of the pose.

## Fire-fly Pose

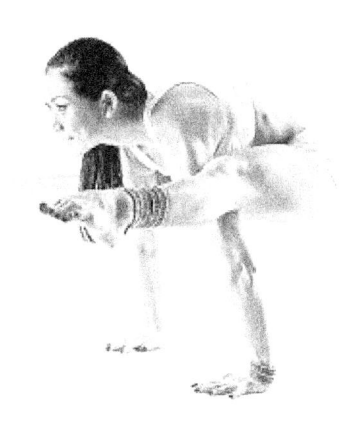

### Steps

- Start by standing upright with your feet a few inches apart and toes slightly pointing out, then bend forward from your hips.

- Slightly bend your knees and bring your right hand through your legs to hold your right calf. Keep your right shoulder behind your right knee.

- Lower your right hand on the floor behind your heel and point your fingers forward.

- Do the same with the left hand.

*Morning Yoga Stretches*

- Open your chest and move it slightly forward, then gently lower your legs until they rest on the backs of your upper arms.

- Lift your feet off the floor and extend them in front of you, so your toes point up toward the ceiling.

- Hold the stretch for a few deep breaths or seconds while focusing on your breath, then release your feet back to the floor.

If you are a beginner and the fire-fly pose seems a bit hard, try doing it this way:

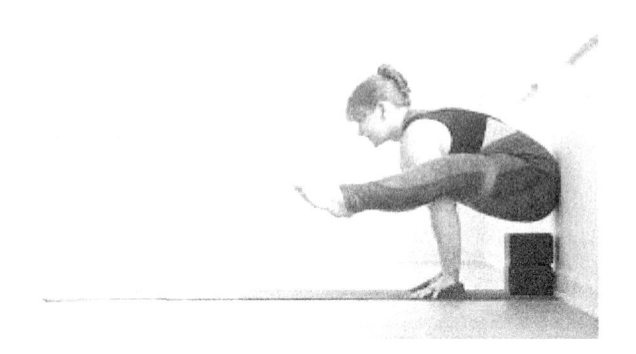

### Steps

- First, get two blocks, bring your mat next to a wall, then stack the blocks horizontally against the wall.

- Stand facing away from the wall with your feet a few inches from it and more than hip-width apart.

- Bend forward from your hips with your knees slightly bent, then bring your hands onto the floor while pressing your buttocks against the wall. Press your palms into the floor with your fingers pointing in front of you.

- Press your buttocks into the wall as you deepen the hip crease and lengthen your spine.

- Lift your legs off the floor and extend them forward, then hold the stretch for a few deep breaths.

# Chapter 7: Morning Yoga Stretches For The Chest

Our chests tend to sink due to prolonged sitting hours doing activities like typing, reading, or carrying heavy stuff; that's why it helps to perform yoga stretches that open the chest.

Try the following stretches:

## Seated Chest Opener

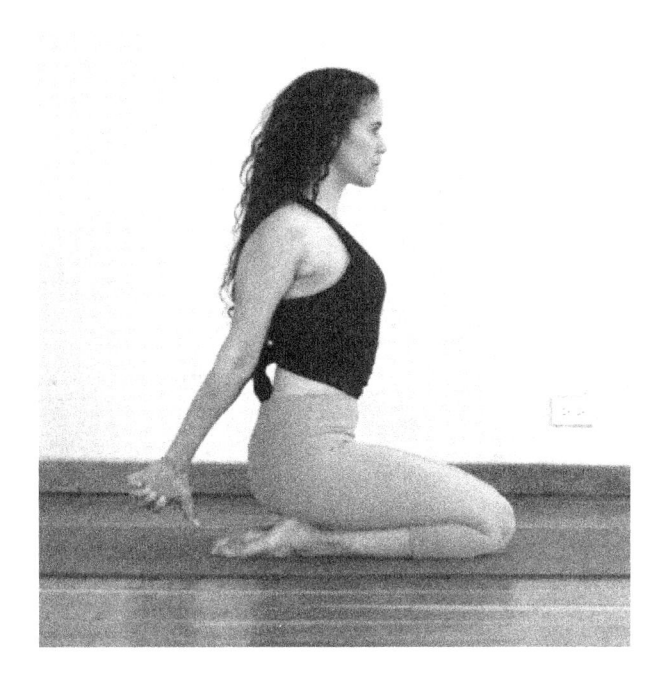

### *Steps*

- Sit comfortably on a mat, cross your legs, or come onto your shins. If you are up on your shins, lay a blanket underneath.

- Lift your arms up toward the ceiling so your ears are between the upper arms.

- Next, lower your arms down by your sides, then interlace your fingers behind you.

*Morning Yoga Stretches*

- Press your shoulders back as you widen your chest. Do not overarch your lower back.

- Hold the pose for a few deep breaths, then release.

## Supported Fish Pose

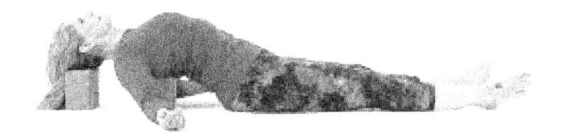

### *Steps*

- Get a dense pillow or two yoga blocks, one taller than the other.

- If using yoga blocks, place the taller one toward the back of your mat and the medium-height block horizontally and about ten inches from the first block. When using the dense pillow, just position it where your back will be.

- Sit on the mat and bend your knees until the soles of your feet are on the floor.

- Position your back on the blocks until the back of your head rests on the tall block and the area in the middle of your shoulder blades, including the tips of your shoulder blades, rests on the second block.

- Bring your arms out to your sides to form a 'T.' Your chest should feel stretched.

- Hold the pose for up to ten deep breaths or five minutes, then return to the sitting position.

## Triceps Stretch

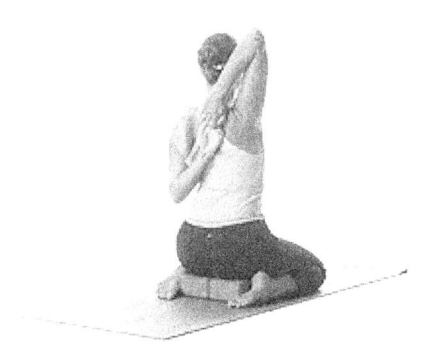

### *Steps*

- Kneel on your mat and place a block lengthways between your feet, then sit on it with your knees still curled and feet behind you.

- Lift your right arm toward the ceiling and bend your elbow. Bring your left hand behind your back and try to interlace your fingers. If interlacing the fingers seems hard, use a strap to help you bring out the pose.

- Lengthen your spine, gaze forward, and stretch your elbows away from each other. Keep your knees and ankles aligned, and do not arch your lower back.

- Hold the pose for 10 deep breaths, then repeat on the other side.

## Thread the Needle

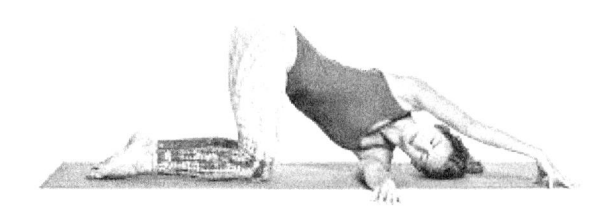

### Steps

- Begin by going down on your knees and hands to have your shoulders above your wrists and hips above the knees. Flex your feet behind you to have the toes face up.

- Lift your right arm up toward the ceiling and extend it as you open your chest toward your right side. Focus your gaze on your right hand.

- Bring your right arm toward your left side by moving it under your chest downward. Your chest should naturally begin to face your right side and torso downward.

- Once your right arm touches the mat, continue to slide it to the right so your right shoulder rests on the mat.

- Stretch your left arm overhead and bring your fingertips to touch the mat. Allow the right side of your head to rest on the mat.

- Hold the pose for ten deep breaths, then repeat on the other side.

*Morning Yoga Stretches*

## Noose Pose

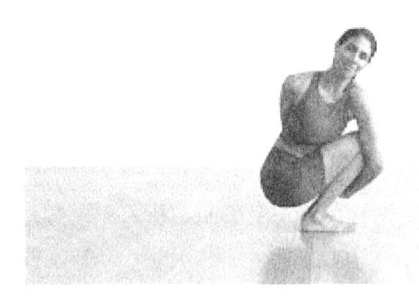

### *Steps*

- Stand upright with your feet together. Bend your knees until you come into a full squat with the toes touching and heels slightly apart. Bring your buttocks to rest on your heels.

- Slightly bring your knees to the left and torso to the right. Bring your shoulder and the back of your left arm toward the outside of the right knee.

- Press your shoulder, left arm, and right knee against each other firmly. Lengthen your torso, making sure it touches the top of your thighs.

- Bring your right arm back, bend at the elbow, and bring your left hand to grab your right wrist.

- Hold this pose for a few deep breaths, then release the twist and repeat on the other side.

*Morning Yoga Stretches*

## Chest Opener With Blocks

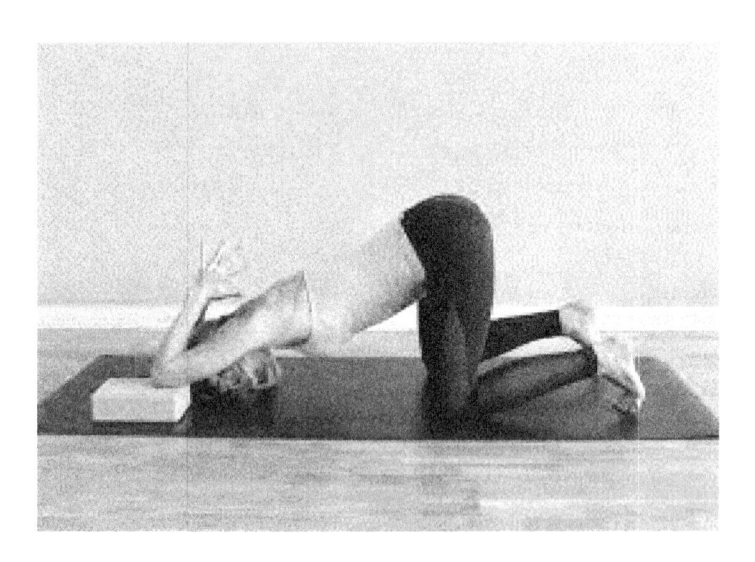

### Steps

- Start by going down on your hands and knees to have your shoulders above your wrists and hips above the knees.

- Place two low blocks under your hands, then bring your elbows to rest on the blocks.

- Lift your hands up toward the ceiling and extend your fingers. Press your palms together with fingers spread and lower your head down until your forehead touches the floor.

- Keep your back straight and the tops of your shoulders in line with the back.

- Hold this pose for ten deep breaths or 30 seconds.

*Morning Yoga Stretches*

# King Cobra Pose

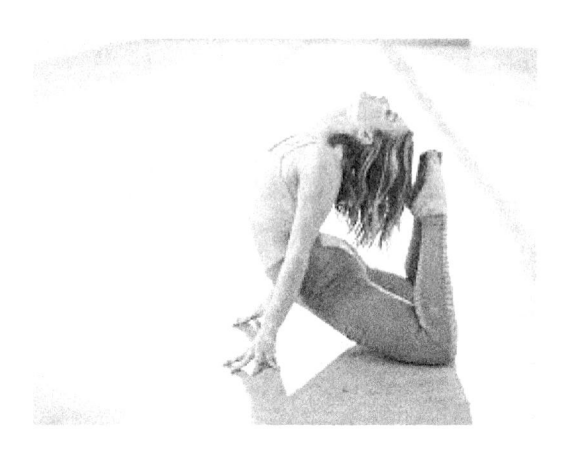

## *Steps*

- Lie on your stomach on your mat and slightly spread your legs.

- Bring your palms onto your mat until they are under your shoulders. Extend your arms as you press your palms into the mat with your fingers spread.

- Open your chest and stretch your neck as you bring your head to look up toward the ceiling.

- Bend your knees as you lift your heels off the floor and toward your head or hips.

- Hold this pose for ten deep breaths, then release.

# Wild Thing

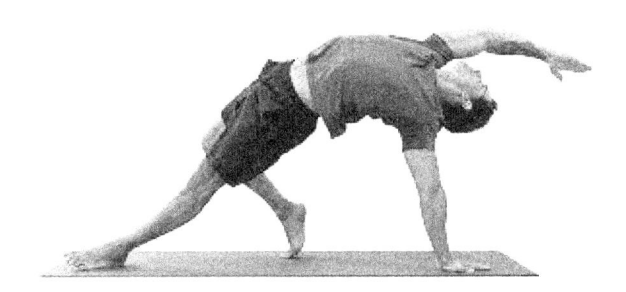

## Steps

- Start with the side plank with your right hand on the floor and underneath your right shoulder. Your body should form a straight line from the shoulders to the toes.

- Tilt your right arm to have the elbow faces the direction of your feet. Lift your left arm toward the ceiling and extend your fingers.

- Lift your left leg and bend at the knee, then place your foot back with your heel raised or toes touching the mat.

*Morning Yoga Stretches*

- Open your chest and rotate it up toward the ceiling. Press your right leg into the mat and rotate your left arm with your palm facing back.

- Extend your left arm overhead while engaging your glutes and direct your gaze up, forward, or downward.

- Hold this pose for a few deep stretches, then come out of the pose.

# Half-frog Pose

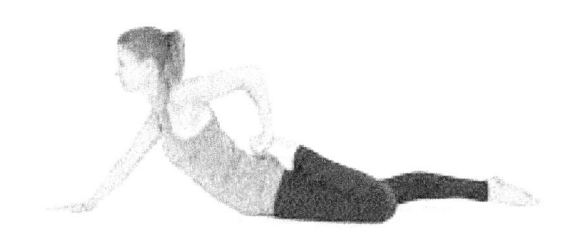

## *Steps*

- Start by lying on your stomach on your mat.

- Bend your elbows until you rest on your forearms. Your shoulders should be above your elbows.

- Squeeze in your abdominals as you cross your right forearm in front of you and bend your left knee until your left foot is up. Bring your right hand behind your back, grab the top of your left foot, then pull it toward your left hip.

*Morning Yoga Stretches*

- Open your chest and keep your gaze forward.
- Hold this pose for 5-10 deep breaths, then release your foot. Repeat the stretch on the other side.

# Conclusion

I wrote this book because I understood that you need mental and physical energy to kickstart your day, and there is no better way to do that than practicing yoga stretches in the morning! As we have already seen, these stretches are a great way to achieve that through their numerous benefits.

I am certain that this book will be of great help to you. Good luck!


PS: I'd like your feedback. If you are happy with this book, please leave a review on Amazon.

Please leave a review for this book on Amazon by visiting the page below:

https://amzn.to/2VMR5qr

Printed in Great Britain
by Amazon